The Role of Nutrition in Mental Health: A Clinical Perspective

Unlocking the Power of Diet to Enhance Mood, Cognition, and Emotional Well-being

By

Dr. M. Qassim

Aug. 2024

Before You Turn the Page… Read This Carefully

- ➢ If you've ever felt that your mood shifts without a clear reason…
- ➢ If your energy crashes, your focus fades, or your mind feels clouded…
- ➢ If anxiety, low mood, or mental fatigue seem to come and go without warning…

There is a high chance that what you eat is quietly influencing how you think, feel, and function.

- ❖ Not in an obvious way.
- ❖ Not in a way most people notice.
- ❖ But in a deep, biological, and powerful way.
- ❖ This book is not about trends, quick fixes, or popular diet myths.

It is about understanding something far more important:

How your daily nutrition shapes your brain chemistry, emotional stability, and mental clarity, often without you realizing it.

Inside these pages, you will begin to see connections you may have never considered before:

- ✓ Why certain foods can stabilize your mood… while others silently disrupt it.
- ✓ How nutrient deficiencies can mimic anxiety, depression, and cognitive decline.
- ✓ Why your gut may be influencing your thoughts more than your mind itself.
- ✓ And how small, precise nutritional changes can lead to measurable mental improvements.

- ➢ This is not about perfection.
- ✓ It is about awareness… and control.
- ✓ Take your time with this book.
- ✓ Let the insights connect.

Because once you understand how nutrition truly affects your mind,
you will never look at food the same way again.

Contents:

Introduction
Understanding the Link Between Nutrition and Mental Health

Something isn't adding up.

You sleep, yet wake up mentally exhausted. You try to stay focused, but your thoughts drift. Your mood shifts without a clear reason, and no matter how much effort you put into managing stress, the results feel inconsistent.

- ➢ Most people are told to look at their mindset, their environment, or their workload.
- ✓ Very few are told to look at what they eat.

Mental health is often treated as something abstract, disconnected from the body. But the reality is far more precise. The brain is not separate from biology. It is shaped, supported, and sometimes disrupted by the nutrients it receives every single day.

What you consume does not just fuel your body. It directly influences brain chemistry, neurotransmitter production, inflammation levels, and cognitive performance.

In recent years, a growing body of research has brought this connection into sharper focus. Nutrients such as vitamins, minerals, amino acids, and essential fatty acids are not optional when it comes to mental stability. They are foundational.

Deficiencies in key elements like vitamin B12, vitamin D, magnesium, and omega-3 fatty acids have been consistently associated with conditions such as depression, anxiety, and cognitive decline. Not as isolated coincidences, but as measurable biological patterns.

This shifts the conversation entirely.

- ✓ Mental health is no longer only about psychology. It is also about physiology.

- ### Purpose and Structure of This Book:
  - ✓ This book was written to bridge a gap that too often remains overlooked.

It is designed for clinicians, dietitians, mental health professionals, and serious readers who want to move beyond general advice and understand the clinical relationship between nutrition and mental health with clarity and depth.

The chapters that follow will guide you through the scientific foundations of nutritional psychiatry, explaining how specific nutrients interact with brain function and emotional regulation. More importantly, the book moves beyond theory.

You will explore practical, evidence-based strategies that integrate nutrition into mental health care, supported by real-world case studies that demonstrate how targeted dietary interventions can produce meaningful change.

- ➢ The goal is not to overwhelm you with information.
- ✓ The goal is to give you clarity.

By the end of this book, you will not only understand how nutrition influences mental health, but you will also be equipped to apply this knowledge with confidence, whether in clinical practice or in your own life.

Because once you see the connection clearly, you cannot unsee it.

And once you understand it, you can start using it.

Chapter 1
The Hidden Science Behind
How Nutrition Shapes Your Mind

You may think your thoughts are entirely your own, but what if your brain chemistry has been quietly shaped by what you eat every single day?

I. <u>The Nervous System and Nutrition:</u>

The nervous system, which includes the brain, spinal cord, and peripheral nerves, is the control center of the body. It regulates thoughts, emotions, and bodily functions. Nutrition plays a fundamental role in maintaining the health and functionality of this complex system. The brain, being the most energy-demanding organ, requires a constant supply of nutrients to function optimally. Key nutrients such as glucose, amino acids, fatty acids, vitamins, and minerals are essential for the growth, repair, and maintenance of neural cells.

Glucose is the primary energy source for the brain. Unlike other organs, the brain cannot store glucose and relies on a continuous supply from the bloodstream. Carbohydrates, which are broken down into glucose, are vital for cognitive functions such as concentration, memory, and learning.

Amino acids, derived from dietary proteins, are the building blocks of neurotransmitters. Neurotransmitters are chemical messengers that transmit signals between neurons. For example, tryptophan, an amino acid found in turkey, eggs, and cheese, is a precursor to serotonin, a neurotransmitter that regulates mood and sleep. Tyrosine, found in dairy products, meats, and nuts, is a precursor to dopamine, which is involved in motivation and reward pathways.

Fatty acids, particularly omega-3 and omega-6 fatty acids, are crucial for brain health. These essential fats, found in fish, nuts, and seeds, are components of cell membranes in the brain. Omega-3 fatty acids, especially docosahexaenoic acid (DHA), support cognitive function and reduce inflammation.

Vitamins and minerals are cofactors in enzymatic reactions involved in neurotransmitter synthesis and energy metabolism. For instance, B vitamins such as B6, B12, and folate are essential for the production of neurotransmitters like serotonin and dopamine. Minerals such as magnesium, zinc, and iron play roles in neuronal signaling and neurotransmitter production.

II.   Neurotransmitters and Hormones:

Neurotransmitters like serotonin, dopamine, and norepinephrine are synthesized from amino acids and are crucial for mood regulation, cognition, and behavior. Serotonin, often called the "feel-good" neurotransmitter, is involved in mood stabilization, feelings of well-being, and happiness. Dopamine is associated with pleasure, motivation, and reward, while norepinephrine affects attention and response to stress.

Hormones, such as cortisol and insulin, also significantly impact mental health. Cortisol, known as the stress hormone, is released during stressful situations and affects mood, motivation, and fear. Prolonged high levels of cortisol can lead to anxiety and depression. Nutrients like omega-3 fatty acids, magnesium, and B vitamins help regulate cortisol levels and support stress management.

Insulin, a hormone that regulates blood sugar levels, is influenced by diet and affects brain function. Fluctuations in blood sugar levels can impact mood and cognitive abilities. A diet balanced in complex carbohydrates, proteins, and healthy fats helps maintain stable blood sugar levels, reducing the risk of mood swings and cognitive impairments.

III.   <u>Key Research Studies:</u>

Numerous studies have explored the connection between nutrition and mental health, providing compelling evidence of the impact of diet on cognitive and emotional well-being.

One landmark study, the SMILES trial (Supporting the Modification of lifestyle in Lowered Emotional States), demonstrated that dietary interventions could significantly reduce symptoms of depression. Participants who followed a Mediterranean-style diet, rich in vegetables, fruits, whole grains, lean proteins, and healthy fats, showed greater improvements in mood compared to those who received social support without dietary changes.

Another significant study published in "The Lancet Psychiatry" highlighted the potential of omega-3 fatty acids in managing depression. The researchers found that individuals with higher intakes of omega-3s had a lower risk of developing depressive symptoms, suggesting these fatty acids play a protective role in mental health.

Research on the gut-brain axis has also shown that gut health profoundly influences mental health. The gut microbiome, a diverse community of microorganisms in the digestive tract, communicates with the brain through neural, endocrine, and immune pathways. Studies have revealed that a healthy gut microbiome, supported by a diet rich in fiber, prebiotics, and probiotics, can positively affect mood, anxiety levels, and cognitive function. For example, a study published in "General Psychiatry" found that participants who consumed a probiotic-rich diet experienced reduced symptoms of anxiety and depression.

- **The Implications of Nutritional Deficiencies:**

Nutritional deficiencies can have detrimental effects on mental health. For example, a deficiency in vitamin B12, commonly found in animal products, can lead to cognitive impairments and mood disorders. Vitamin B12 is essential for the production of red blood cells and the maintenance of nerve cells. Its deficiency can cause symptoms such as fatigue, memory loss, and depression.

Low levels of vitamin D, synthesized in the skin upon exposure to sunlight and found in certain foods like fatty fish and fortified dairy products, have been associated with an increased risk of depression and anxiety. Vitamin D receptors are present in the brain, and its deficiency can impair cognitive function and mood regulation.

Iron deficiency, prevalent among women and vegetarians, can cause fatigue, cognitive impairments, and mood disturbances. Iron is crucial for the production of hemoglobin, which transports oxygen to the brain. Low iron levels can result in reduced oxygen delivery, affecting cognitive function and emotional well-being.

Addressing these deficiencies through dietary changes or supplementation can significantly improve mental health outcomes. For instance, increasing the intake of iron-rich foods like lean meats, legumes, and leafy greens can alleviate symptoms of iron deficiency anemia and its associated cognitive and emotional effects. Similarly, supplementing with vitamin D during the winter months or for individuals with limited sun exposure can help maintain optimal levels and support mental health.

- **The Role of Antioxidants:**

Antioxidants play a crucial role in protecting the brain from oxidative stress, a condition where there is an imbalance between free radicals and antioxidants in the body. Oxidative stress can damage brain cells, leading to cognitive decline and mental health disorders. Nutrients such as vitamins C and E, selenium, and flavonoids found in colorful fruits and vegetables have potent antioxidant properties that help neutralize free radicals and support brain health.

Vitamin C, found in citrus fruits, strawberries, and bell peppers, is a powerful antioxidant that protects the brain from oxidative damage and supports the immune system. Vitamin E, present in nuts, seeds, and green leafy vegetables, helps protect cell membranes from oxidative damage and supports cognitive function.

Selenium, found in Brazil nuts, seafood, and whole grains, is a trace mineral that plays a vital role in antioxidant defense and thyroid function. Flavonoids, present in berries, tea, and dark chocolate, have anti-inflammatory and antioxidant properties that support brain health and cognitive function.

In conclusion, the intricate relationship between nutrition and mental health underscores the importance of a balanced diet in maintaining and improving mental well-being. Understanding how nutrients affect the nervous system, neurotransmitters, and hormones helps us make informed dietary choices that promote mental health. The following chapters will delve deeper into specific nutrients and dietary patterns, offering practical strategies for integrating nutrition into mental health care.

<u>Conclusion:</u>

This chapter has provided a comprehensive overview of the science behind nutrition and mental health. By exploring the roles of the nervous system, neurotransmitters, hormones, and key research studies, we have highlighted the significant impact of diet on mental well-being. Nutritional deficiencies and the protective role of antioxidants have also been discussed, emphasizing the need for a balanced diet to support optimal brain function.

As we move forward, the next chapters will focus on the detailed examination of macronutrients and micronutrients, the gut-brain connection, and specific dietary patterns that influence mental health. Practical strategies for managing mental health conditions through nutrition will be provided, along with real-life case studies and guidelines for clinicians. Through this journey, we aim to empower readers with the knowledge and tools to make informed dietary choices that enhance mental well-being and overall health.

Chapter 2
How Proteins, Carbs, and Fats Quietly Control Your Mood and Brain Function

Before you blame stress or life circumstances, it's worth asking a simpler question: **what have you been feeding your brain?**

I. <u>Proteins and Brain Health:</u>

- **Essential Role of Proteins:**

- Proteins are fundamental for numerous bodily functions, especially for brain health. They consist of amino acids, which are the building blocks for neurotransmitters, the chemical messengers that transmit signals within the brain and throughout the nervous system.

- Neurotransmitters such as serotonin, dopamine, and norepinephrine are synthesized from amino acids. These neurotransmitters play critical roles in regulating mood, cognition, and overall mental health. For instance, serotonin influences mood and anxiety, dopamine affects pleasure and motivation, and norepinephrine is involved in the body's stress response.

- **Amino Acids and Neurotransmitters:**
  - **Tryptophan and Serotonin:**

Tryptophan is an essential amino acid that serves as a precursor to serotonin. Serotonin is a neurotransmitter that regulates mood, sleep, and appetite. Consuming foods high in tryptophan, such as turkey, chicken, milk, cheese, yogurt, nuts, and seeds, can increase serotonin levels in the brain, potentially improving mood and promoting a sense of well-being.

o **Tyrosine and Dopamine:**

Tyrosine, a non-essential amino acid, is a precursor to dopamine, which is involved in motivation, pleasure, and reward. Foods rich in tyrosine, including eggs, dairy products, meat, fish, soy products, and legumes, can support dopamine production, enhancing cognitive function and emotional stability.

- **Protein Deficiency and Cognitive Function:**
- Inadequate protein intake can lead to deficiencies in essential amino acids, resulting in impaired cognitive function, mood disorders, and reduced mental performance. Symptoms of protein deficiency may include mental fatigue, difficulty concentrating, depression, anxiety, and irritability.
- Ensuring adequate protein intake is crucial for maintaining optimal brain function and mental health. Dietary sources of high-quality proteins include lean meats, fish, dairy products, eggs, legumes, nuts, and seeds.

II. <u>Carbohydrates and Mood:</u>

- **Energy Source for the Brain:**

Carbohydrates are the brain's primary energy source. When consumed, carbohydrates are broken down into glucose, which fuels brain activity. The brain relies heavily on a steady supply of glucose to function properly, making carbohydrate intake critical for mental health.

- **Types of Carbohydrates:**
  - **Complex Carbohydrates:**
- Found in whole grains, vegetables, legumes, and fruits, complex carbohydrates provide a slow and steady release of glucose into the bloodstream. This helps maintain stable energy levels and mood throughout the day.
- Foods such as whole grain bread, brown rice, quinoa, sweet potatoes, and leafy greens are excellent sources of complex carbohydrates.
  - **Simple Carbohydrates:**
- Found in sugary foods and drinks, simple carbohydrates cause rapid spikes and crashes in blood sugar levels, leading to mood swings, irritability, and energy fluctuations.
- Examples of simple carbohydrates include sweets, pastries, sugary drinks, and refined grains.

- **Glycemic Index and Mood Regulation:**
- The glycemic index (GI) measures how quickly foods raise blood glucose levels. Foods with a low GI release glucose slowly into the bloodstream, promoting stable energy levels and reducing the risk of mood disorders.
- Incorporating low-GI foods like oats, barley, lentils, apples, and carrots into the diet can support mental well-being by preventing blood sugar fluctuations and associated mood swings.

III.   <u>Healthy Fats and Cognitive Function:</u>

- **Importance of Healthy Fats:**

   Fats are essential for brain health. The brain is composed of approximately 60% fat, and healthy fats support the structure and function of brain cells. Fats are involved in the formation of cell membranes, the production of myelin (which insulates nerve fibers), and the regulation of inflammation and neurotransmitter function.

- **Types of Healthy Fats:**
  - **Omega-3 Fatty Acids:**
- Found in fatty fish (such as salmon, mackerel, and sardines), flaxseeds, chia seeds, walnuts, and algae, omega-3 fatty acids are critical for cognitive function and emotional regulation. They reduce inflammation, support neurotransmitter function, and protect against neurodegenerative diseases.
- Omega-3 fatty acids, particularly EPA and DHA, have been shown to improve mood, reduce symptoms of depression, and enhance cognitive performance.
  - **Monounsaturated Fats:**
- Found in olive oil, avocados, nuts, and seeds, monounsaturated fats support brain health by reducing oxidative stress and inflammation. These fats can improve brain plasticity, enhance learning and memory, and protect against age-related cognitive decline.

  - **Polyunsaturated Fats:**
- In addition to omega-3s, polyunsaturated fats include omega-6 fatty acids found in vegetable oils, nuts, and seeds. While necessary, it is important to balance omega-6 intake with omega-3s to prevent excessive inflammation.

- **Effects of Fat Deficiency on the Brain:**
- A diet low in healthy fats can impair cognitive function, increase the risk of depression, and affect overall brain health. Symptoms of fat deficiency may include difficulty concentrating, memory problems, mood swings, and increased susceptibility to stress.
- Ensuring adequate intake of healthy fats is crucial for maintaining mental well-being and supporting brain function.

- **Balancing Macronutrients for Optimal Mental Health:**
  - **Proportional Intake:**
- Balancing proteins, carbohydrates, and fats is essential for supporting mental health. Each macronutrient plays a unique role, and an imbalance can lead to nutritional deficiencies and mental health issues.
- A well-balanced diet that includes a variety of nutrient-dense foods can provide the necessary macronutrients for optimal brain function and emotional stability.
  - **Personalized Nutrition:**
- Individual nutritional needs vary based on factors such as age, gender, activity level, and health status. Personalized nutrition plans can help optimize mental health by addressing specific dietary requirements and preferences.
- Working with a healthcare provider or nutritionist can ensure that dietary plans are tailored to meet individual needs, promoting overall well-being.

Conclusion:

Macronutrients play a vital role in mental health, influencing brain function, mood, and cognitive performance. Proteins provide the building blocks for neurotransmitters, carbohydrates supply the brain with energy, and healthy fats support brain structure and function. Understanding the impact of macronutrients on mental health can help individuals make informed dietary choices to support their well-being. By balancing protein, carbohydrate, and fat intake, and focusing on nutrient-dense foods, we can enhance our mental health and overall quality of life. This chapter provides a foundation for exploring the specific roles of micronutrients in mental health, which will be covered in the next chapter.

Chapter 3
The Essential Vitamins and Minerals
Your Brain Cannot Function Without

Sometimes, what feels like emotional instability is not psychological at all, it's biological, and often missing something small but critical.

I. **<u>Essential Vitamins:</u>**

- **Vitamin B Complex:**
  - **Vitamin B1 (Thiamine):**
    - ❖ **Role and Importance:**
- Thiamine is crucial for converting carbohydrates into energy, which is essential for brain function. It plays a significant role in glucose metabolism, providing the brain with the energy it needs to function optimally.
- Thiamine is involved in the synthesis of neurotransmitters, particularly acetylcholine, which is important for memory and learning.
    - ❖ **Deficiency Symptoms:**
- Deficiency can lead to mental fatigue, irritability, poor concentration, and memory problems. Severe deficiency can cause Wernicke-Korsakoff syndrome, a serious brain disorder.
- **Sources:** Whole grains, legumes, nuts, pork, and fortified cereals.
  - **Vitamin B6 (Pyridoxine):**
    - ❖ **Role and Importance:**
- B6 is vital for the synthesis of neurotransmitters such as serotonin, dopamine, and GABA, which are crucial for mood regulation and mental health.

- It also plays a role in the production of melatonin, which regulates sleep patterns.

❖ **Deficiency Symptoms:**

- Deficiency can result in mood disturbances, irritability, confusion, and cognitive decline. It is also linked to symptoms of depression and anxiety.
- **Sources:** Poultry, fish, potatoes, bananas, chickpeas, and fortified cereals.

o **Vitamin B9 (Folate):**

❖ **Role and Importance:**

- Folate is essential for DNA synthesis and repair, and it plays a critical role in the production of neurotransmitters.
- It helps in the formation of red blood cells and is vital for brain development and function.

❖ **Deficiency Symptoms:**

- Folate deficiency can lead to symptoms of depression, cognitive impairment, and fatigue. It is also associated with an increased risk of neural tube defects in unborn babies.
- **Sources:** Leafy greens, legumes, nuts, seeds, and fortified cereals.

o **Vitamin B12 (Cobalamin):**

❖ **Role and Importance:**

- B12 is crucial for the maintenance of the nervous system and the formation of red blood cells. It is involved in the production of DNA and the metabolism of every cell in the body.
- It helps in the synthesis of myelin, the protective sheath around nerves, and the production of neurotransmitters.

❖ **Deficiency Symptoms:**

- Deficiency can lead to memory loss, mood changes, cognitive decline, and neurological issues such as numbness and tingling.
- **Sources:** Meat, dairy products, eggs, fish, and fortified cereals.

- o **Vitamin D:**
  - ❖ **Role and Importance:**
- Vitamin D receptors are present in the brain, and it plays a role in brain development and function. It helps regulate the immune system and reduce inflammation.
- Vitamin D is involved in the production of neurotransmitters and the protection of neurons.
  - ❖ **Deficiency Symptoms:**
- Low levels of vitamin D are associated with mood disorders such as depression and anxiety. Deficiency can also lead to cognitive impairment and increased risk of neurodegenerative diseases.
- **Sources:** Sunlight exposure, fatty fish (such as salmon and mackerel), fortified dairy products, and supplements.
- **Vitamin C (Ascorbic Acid):**
  - ❖ **Role and Importance:**
- Vitamin C is a powerful antioxidant that protects the brain from oxidative stress. It is involved in the synthesis of neurotransmitters such as dopamine and serotonin.
- It helps in the formation of collagen, which is necessary for the maintenance of blood vessels in the brain.
  - ❖ **Deficiency Symptoms:**
- Deficiency can lead to fatigue, depression, and cognitive decline. Severe deficiency can cause scurvy, which includes symptoms such as weakness, anemia, and gum disease.
- **Sources:** Citrus fruits, strawberries, bell peppers, broccoli, Brussels sprouts, and tomatoes.

II. <u>Critical Minerals:</u>

- **Magnesium:**
  - ❖ **Role and Importance:**
- Magnesium is involved in over 300 biochemical reactions in the body, including those related to brain function. It helps regulate neurotransmitter activity and reduce inflammation.
- It plays a role in the synthesis of serotonin and the function of GABA receptors, which are important for mood regulation and relaxation.
  - ❖ **Deficiency Symptoms:**
- Deficiency can lead to symptoms such as anxiety, depression, irritability, fatigue, and insomnia. It is also associated with an increased risk of migraines and ADHD.
- **Sources:** Dark leafy greens, nuts, seeds, whole grains, fish, and avocados.

- **Zinc:**
  - ❖ **Role and Importance:**
- Zinc is crucial for brain function and neuroplasticity. It is involved in the regulation of neurotransmitters and the protection of neurons from oxidative stress.
- It plays a role in the growth and repair of brain cells and the formation of new neural connections.

  - ❖ **Deficiency Symptoms:**
- Deficiency can result in symptoms such as depression, anxiety, irritability, cognitive impairment, and weakened immune function.
- **Sources:** Meat, shellfish, legumes, seeds, nuts, dairy products, and whole grains.

- **Iron:**
  - ❖ **Role and Importance:**
- Iron is essential for the production of hemoglobin, which transports oxygen to the brain. It is involved in the synthesis of neurotransmitters and myelin.
- Adequate iron levels are necessary for maintaining energy levels and cognitive function.
  - ❖ **Deficiency Symptoms:**
- Iron deficiency can lead to symptoms such as fatigue, poor concentration, memory problems, irritability, and anemia. Severe deficiency can cause cognitive and developmental delays in children.
- **Sources:** Red meat, poultry, fish, legumes, lentils, spinach, and fortified cereals.

- **Calcium:**
  - ❖ **Role and Importance:**
- Calcium is vital for neurotransmitter release and nerve function. It plays a role in muscle contraction, including the heart, and is necessary for the transmission of signals in the nervous system.
- It helps regulate the release of neurotransmitters and supports synaptic plasticity, which is important for learning and memory.

  - ❖ **Deficiency Symptoms:**
- Deficiency can lead to symptoms such as muscle cramps, irritability, anxiety, depression, and increased risk of osteoporosis.
- **Sources:** Dairy products, leafy greens, fortified plant-based milks, tofu, and almonds.

III.   <u>Micronutrient Deficiencies:</u>

- **Identifying Deficiencies:**
- Common symptoms of micronutrient deficiencies include fatigue, mood swings, cognitive decline, decreased immune function, and various physical symptoms depending on the specific deficiency.
- Nutrient deficiencies often result from poor dietary choices, chronic illnesses, or absorption issues. Conditions like celiac disease, Crohn's disease, and certain medications can interfere with nutrient absorption.

- **Addressing Deficiencies:**
  - **Dietary Changes:**
- Improving diet quality by incorporating a variety of nutrient-dense foods can help prevent and address micronutrient deficiencies. A balanced diet rich in fruits, vegetables, whole grains, lean proteins, and healthy fats is essential.
  - **Supplementation:**
- In cases of severe deficiency or absorption issues, supplementation may be necessary. It is important to consult a healthcare provider before starting any supplement regimen to ensure proper dosage and prevent toxicity.
- Regular monitoring and follow-up are essential to ensure that nutrient levels are optimized and maintained over time. Blood tests and dietary assessments can help track progress and adjust interventions as needed.

Conclusion:

Micronutrients, including essential vitamins and minerals, play a pivotal role in maintaining mental health and cognitive function. Vitamins such as the B complex, D, and C, and minerals like magnesium, zinc, iron, and calcium, contribute to neurotransmitter production, brain function, and mood regulation. Understanding and addressing micronutrient deficiencies through dietary changes and supplementation can significantly improve mental well-being. This chapter provides a comprehensive overview of the importance of micronutrients, setting the stage for the next chapter, which will explore the gut-brain connection and its impact on mental health.

Chapter 4
The Gut-Brain Connection: How Your Microbiome Influences Your Thoughts and Emotions

There is a conversation happening inside your body right now, between your gut and your brain, and it may be shaping how you feel more than you realize.

I. <u>Understanding the Gut-Brain Axis:</u>

- **The Bidirectional Communication System:**
  - **Role and Importance:**
- The gut-brain axis is a complex communication network linking the central nervous system (CNS) with the enteric nervous system (ENS) in the gastrointestinal tract. This bidirectional communication system involves neural, hormonal, and immunological signaling pathways.
- The vagus nerve, a major component of the parasympathetic nervous system, plays a critical role in transmitting signals between the gut and the brain.
  - **Impact on Mental Health:**
- The gut-brain axis influences mood, cognition, and mental health. Disruptions in this communication can contribute to various psychiatric and neurological disorders, such as anxiety, depression, autism, and neurodegenerative diseases.
- Stress and emotional disturbances can affect gut function, leading to conditions like irritable bowel syndrome (IBS) and inflammatory bowel disease (IBD).

- **Microbiome Composition and Function:**
  - **Role and Importance:**
- The gut microbiome consists of trillions of microorganisms, including bacteria, viruses, fungi, and other microbes. These microorganisms play a crucial role in digestion, immune function, and overall health.
- The composition and diversity of the gut microbiome are influenced by diet, lifestyle, genetics, and environmental factors.
  - **Impact on Mental Health:**
- The gut microbiome produces neurotransmitters such as serotonin, dopamine, and GABA, which are important for mood regulation and cognitive function.
- Dysbiosis, an imbalance in the gut microbiome, is associated with various mental health disorders, including depression, anxiety, and autism spectrum disorders.

## II.	Probiotics and Mental Health:

- **Role and Importance:**
- Probiotics are live microorganisms that confer health benefits when consumed in adequate amounts. They can help restore and maintain a healthy gut microbiome.
- Probiotics produce short-chain fatty acids (SCFAs) and other metabolites that have anti-inflammatory and neuroprotective effects.
- Probiotics can enhance the production of neurotransmitters and modulate the immune response, thereby influencing brain function and mental health.

- **Scientific Evidence:**
  - **Clinical Studies:**
- Numerous clinical studies have shown that probiotics can reduce symptoms of depression and anxiety. For example, Lactobacillus and Bifidobacterium strains have been found to improve mood and cognitive function in both healthy individuals and those with psychiatric disorders.
- Probiotic supplementation has been shown to reduce inflammation and oxidative stress, which are linked to mental health disorders.
  - **Mechanisms of Action:**
- Probiotics influence the gut-brain axis through various mechanisms, including modulation of the immune system, production of neurotransmitters, and enhancement of gut barrier function.

III. <u>Dietary Strategies for a Healthy Microbiome:</u>

- **Prebiotics and Fiber:**
  - **Role and Importance:**
- Prebiotics are non-digestible fibers that stimulate the growth and activity of beneficial gut bacteria. They serve as food for probiotics and help maintain a balanced gut microbiome.
- High-fiber diets promote the production of SCFAs, which have anti-inflammatory and neuroprotective effects.
  - **Sources:**
- Prebiotic-rich foods include garlic, onions, leeks, asparagus, bananas, oats, and legumes.
- Dietary fiber is found in fruits, vegetables, whole grains, nuts, and seeds.

- o **Impact on Mental Health:**
- Prebiotic supplementation has been shown to reduce stress, anxiety, and depressive symptoms. It also improves cognitive function and overall mental well-being.

- • **Fermented Foods:**
  - o **Role and Importance:**
- Fermented foods contain live beneficial bacteria that can enhance the gut microbiome. They provide a natural source of probiotics and improve gut health.
  - o **Sources:**
- Common fermented foods include yogurt, kefir, sauerkraut, kimchi, miso, tempeh, and kombucha.
  - o **Impact on Mental Health:**
- Regular consumption of fermented foods has been associated with reduced symptoms of anxiety and depression. It also supports cognitive function and emotional resilience.

- • **Balanced Diet:**
  - o **Role and Importance:**
- A balanced diet rich in whole foods, diverse plant-based foods, and healthy fats supports a healthy gut microbiome. It provides essential nutrients that promote gut and brain health.
  - o **Impact on Mental Health:**
- Diets high in processed foods, sugar, and unhealthy fats can negatively impact the gut microbiome and contribute to mental health disorders. Conversely, a nutrient-rich diet can enhance mental well-being and cognitive function.

- **Lifestyle Factors:**
  - **Stress Management:**
- Chronic stress can disrupt the gut microbiome and impair gut-brain communication. Stress management techniques such as mindfulness, meditation, yoga, and regular exercise can improve gut health and mental well-being.
  - **Sleep and Circadian Rhythms:**
- Adequate sleep and maintaining regular circadian rhythms are crucial for gut and brain health. Disrupted sleep patterns can negatively affect the gut microbiome and contribute to mental health issues.
  - **Physical Activity:**
- Regular physical activity promotes a healthy gut microbiome and enhances mental health. Exercise stimulates the production of beneficial gut bacteria and reduces inflammation.

Conclusion:

The gut-brain connection plays a pivotal role in mental health, with the gut microbiome significantly influencing brain function and mood regulation. Understanding the bidirectional communication between the gut and the brain, and the role of probiotics and dietary strategies in maintaining a healthy microbiome, is crucial for mental well-being. This chapter highlights the importance of a balanced diet, prebiotics, probiotics, and lifestyle factors in supporting the gut-brain axis. By optimizing gut health, individuals can improve their mental health and overall quality of life. The next chapter will explore how different dietary patterns impact mental health, providing further insights into the relationship between diet and psychological well-being.

Chapter 5
Dietary Patterns That Can Strengthen or Sabotage Your Mental Health

It's not just what you eat once in a while that matters, it's the pattern you repeat without thinking that defines how your mind performs.

I.   <u>Mediterranean Diet:</u>

- **Overview:**
- The Mediterranean diet is characterized by high consumption of fruits, vegetables, whole grains, legumes, nuts, seeds, olive oil, and moderate consumption of fish and poultry. It includes low to moderate amounts of dairy and red wine, and limited intake of red meat and processed foods.

- **Nutrient Composition:**
- Rich in healthy fats (especially omega-3 fatty acids), antioxidants, vitamins, minerals, and fiber.

- **Impact on Mental Health:**
  - **Research Evidence:**
- Studies have shown that adherence to the Mediterranean diet is associated with lower risks of depression, anxiety, and cognitive decline. This diet promotes brain health by reducing inflammation and oxidative stress, and enhancing neuroplasticity.
- The PREDIMED study demonstrated that individuals following the Mediterranean diet supplemented with nuts or olive oil had a lower incidence of depression compared to those on a control diet.

    o **Mechanisms of Action:**
- The diet's anti-inflammatory properties and high content of antioxidants (such as polyphenols in olive oil and resveratrol in red wine) protect against neuroinflammation and oxidative damage.
- Omega-3 fatty acids from fish and plant sources support the structural integrity of brain cell membranes and facilitate neurotransmission.

    o **Practical Tips:**
- Incorporate a variety of colorful fruits and vegetables into daily meals.
- Choose whole grains over refined grains.
- Use olive oil as the primary fat source for cooking and dressings.
- Include fatty fish such as salmon, mackerel, and sardines in the diet at least twice a week.
- Snack on nuts and seeds, and include legumes in soups, salads, and main dishes.

II.   <u>Plant-Based Diets:</u>

- **Overview:**
- Plant-based diets emphasize the consumption of whole plant foods such as fruits, vegetables, legumes, nuts, seeds, and whole grains, while minimizing or eliminating animal products.
- **Nutrient Composition:**
- High in fiber, antioxidants, vitamins (especially C, E, and folate), minerals, and phytonutrients. Typically lower in saturated fat and cholesterol.
- **Impact on Mental Health:**
- o **Research Evidence:**
- Plant-based diets are associated with lower rates of depression and anxiety. They may also reduce the risk of cognitive decline and neurodegenerative diseases.

- Studies have found that individuals who follow vegetarian or vegan diets report better mood and lower levels of stress and anxiety compared to omnivores.
  - o **Mechanisms of Action:**
- High fiber content promotes a healthy gut microbiome, which positively influences the gut-brain axis.
- Abundance of antioxidants and phytonutrients helps reduce inflammation and oxidative stress, protecting brain cells.
- Folate and other B vitamins in plant-based diets support neurotransmitter synthesis and function.
  - o **Practical Tips:**
- Focus on whole, minimally processed plant foods.
- Ensure adequate intake of protein from legumes, nuts, seeds, and soy products.
- Consider fortified foods or supplements for nutrients that may be low in plant-based diets, such as vitamin B12, vitamin D, and omega-3 fatty acids.
- Experiment with a variety of plant-based recipes to keep meals interesting and nutritionally balanced.

III. <u>Western Diet and Mental Health:</u>

- **Overview:**
- The Western diet is characterized by high consumption of processed and refined foods, red and processed meats, sugary beverages, and high-fat dairy products. It often includes large amounts of saturated fats, trans fats, sugars, and salt.
- **Nutrient Composition:**
- High in calories, unhealthy fats, refined sugars, and sodium. Low in fiber, antioxidants, vitamins, and minerals.

- **Impact on Mental Health:**
  - **Research Evidence:**
- The Western diet is associated with higher risks of depression, anxiety, and cognitive decline. It contributes to systemic inflammation, oxidative stress, and metabolic disorders, all of which negatively impact brain health.
- Studies have found that individuals who consume a Western diet are more likely to experience mood disorders and poorer cognitive performance.
  - **Mechanisms of Action:**
- High levels of refined sugars and unhealthy fats can lead to insulin resistance and inflammation, which adversely affect brain function.
- Deficiency in essential nutrients (such as omega-3 fatty acids, vitamins, and minerals) impairs neurotransmitter production and brain health.
- Processed foods often contain additives and preservatives that may have neurotoxic effects.
  - **Practical Tips:**
- Reduce the intake of processed and fast foods.
- Limit the consumption of sugary beverages and snacks.
- Opt for whole foods and home-cooked meals made from fresh ingredients.
- Gradually replace unhealthy fats with healthier options like olive oil, avocados, and nuts.

Conclusion:

Dietary patterns have a profound impact on mental health. The Mediterranean and plant-based diets are associated with numerous benefits for brain function and emotional well-being, primarily due to their rich nutrient profiles and anti-inflammatory properties. In contrast, the Western diet, high in processed foods and unhealthy fats, is linked to increased risks of mood disorders and cognitive decline. By adopting healthy dietary patterns and making informed food choices, individuals can support their mental health and improve overall quality of life. The next chapter will delve into specific nutrition strategies for managing depression and anxiety, providing practical guidance for dietary interventions to alleviate these common mental health conditions.

Chapter 6
Targeted Nutrition Strategies to Manage Depression and Anxiety Naturally

When your mood feels out of control, the solution may not always be more effort, but a different kind of input.

I. <u>Dietary Approaches for Depression:</u>

- **The Role of Nutrients:**
  - **Omega-3 Fatty Acids:**
    - ❖ **Role and Importance:**
- Omega-3 fatty acids, particularly EPA and DHA, are essential for brain health. They support cell membrane fluidity and neurotransmitter function, which are crucial for mood regulation.
    - ❖ **Sources:**
- Fatty fish (such as salmon, mackerel, and sardines), flaxseeds, chia seeds, walnuts, and fish oil supplements.
    - ❖ **Research Evidence:**
- Numerous studies have shown that higher intake of omega-3 fatty acids is associated with lower rates of depression. Supplementation with EPA and DHA has been found to reduce depressive symptoms, particularly in individuals with low baseline levels.
  - **B Vitamins:**
    - ❖ **Role and Importance:**
- B vitamins, including B6, B9 (folate), and B12, play key roles in neurotransmitter synthesis and function. They are crucial for the production of serotonin, dopamine, and other mood-regulating chemicals.

❖ **Sources:**
- Whole grains, legumes, leafy greens, eggs, dairy products, and fortified cereals.
  ❖ **Research Evidence:**
- Deficiencies in B vitamins are linked to an increased risk of depression. Supplementation with these vitamins has been shown to improve mood and reduce depressive symptoms, particularly in individuals with deficiencies.
  o **Magnesium:**
    ❖ **Role and Importance:**
- Magnesium is involved in numerous biochemical reactions in the brain, including neurotransmitter release and neural plasticity. It helps regulate stress responses and promotes relaxation.
  ❖ **Sources:**
- Dark leafy greens, nuts, seeds, whole grains, and legumes.
  ❖ **Research Evidence:**
- Low magnesium levels are associated with an increased risk of depression. Supplementation has been found to reduce symptoms of depression, particularly in individuals with low dietary intake.
  o **Vitamin D:**
    ❖ **Role and Importance:**
- Vitamin D receptors are present in the brain, and this vitamin plays a role in brain development and function. It also modulates the immune system and reduces inflammation.
  ❖ **Sources:**
- Sunlight exposure, fatty fish, fortified dairy products, and supplements.
  ❖ **Research Evidence:**
- Low levels of vitamin D are linked to higher rates of depression. Supplementation with vitamin D has been shown to improve mood

and alleviate depressive symptoms, particularly in individuals with deficiencies.

- **Dietary Patterns:**
  - **Mediterranean Diet:**
    - ❖ **Key Components:**
- High consumption of fruits, vegetables, whole grains, legumes, nuts, seeds, and olive oil, with moderate intake of fish and poultry, and low intake of red meat and processed foods.
    - ❖ **Impact on Depression:**
- The anti-inflammatory and antioxidant properties of the Mediterranean diet help protect against neuroinflammation and oxidative stress, which are linked to depression. Studies have shown that adherence to this diet is associated with a lower risk of depression and improved mood.
  - **Anti-Inflammatory Diet:**
    - ❖ **Key Components:**
- Emphasis on foods with anti-inflammatory properties, such as fruits, vegetables, whole grains, fatty fish, nuts, seeds, and olive oil. Avoidance of processed foods, refined sugars, and trans fats.
    - ❖ **Impact on Depression:**
- Chronic inflammation is linked to the development of depression. An anti-inflammatory diet can help reduce inflammation and improve mood by providing a rich source of antioxidants, omega-3 fatty acids, and other anti-inflammatory nutrients.

II. **<u>Anxiety and Nutrition:</u>**

- **The Role of Nutrients:**
  - **GABA (Gamma-Aminobutyric Acid):**
    - ❖ **Role and Importance:**

- GABA is a neurotransmitter that promotes relaxation and reduces anxiety by inhibiting neural activity.
    - ❖ **Sources:**
- Fermented foods (such as yogurt, kefir, and tempeh), green tea, and certain fruits and vegetables.
    - ❖ **Research Evidence:**
- Increasing GABA levels through diet and supplementation has been shown to reduce symptoms of anxiety and promote relaxation.
  - **Magnesium:**
    - ❖ **Role and Importance:**
- Magnesium helps regulate the body's stress response and promotes relaxation by modulating the activity of the hypothalamic-pituitary-adrenal (HPA) axis.
    - ❖ **Sources:**
- Dark leafy greens, nuts, seeds, whole grains, and legumes.
    - ❖ **Research Evidence:**
- Low magnesium levels are associated with higher levels of anxiety. Supplementation has been found to reduce symptoms of anxiety, particularly in individuals with low dietary intake.
  - **Omega-3 Fatty Acids:**
    - ❖ **Role and Importance:**
- Omega-3 fatty acids help reduce inflammation and support brain function, which can alleviate symptoms of anxiety.
    - ❖ **Sources:**
- Fatty fish, flaxseeds, chia seeds, walnuts, and fish oil supplements.

❖ **Research Evidence:**

- Higher intake of omega-3 fatty acids is associated with lower levels of anxiety. Supplementation with EPA and DHA has been found to reduce symptoms of anxiety, particularly in individuals with high levels of inflammation.

  o **Probiotics:**

  ❖ **Role and Importance:**

- Probiotics support a healthy gut microbiome, which can influence the gut-brain axis and reduce symptoms of anxiety.

  ❖ **Sources:**

- Fermented foods (such as yogurt, kefir, sauerkraut, and kimchi) and probiotic supplements.

  ❖ **Research Evidence:**

- Probiotic supplementation has been shown to reduce symptoms of anxiety and improve mood by modulating the gut-brain axis.

- **Dietary Patterns:**
  o **Anti-Anxiety Diet:**

  ❖ **Key Components:**

- Emphasis on nutrient-dense foods that support brain function and reduce inflammation, such as fruits, vegetables, whole grains, lean proteins, and healthy fats. Avoidance of processed foods, refined sugars, and caffeine.

  ❖ **Impact on Anxiety:**

- A diet rich in anti-inflammatory and mood-regulating nutrients can help reduce symptoms of anxiety by supporting brain function and reducing stress.

- o **Mindfulness-Based Eating:**
  - ❖ **Key Components:**
- Focus on mindful eating practices, such as eating slowly, savoring each bite, and paying attention to hunger and fullness cues.
  - ❖ **Impact on Anxiety:**
- Mindful eating can help reduce symptoms of anxiety by promoting relaxation, reducing stress, and improving the overall relationship with food.

III. <u>Case Studies:</u>

- o **Case Study 1: Addressing Depression with the Mediterranean Diet:**
  - ❖ **Background:**
- A 45-year-old woman with a history of major depressive disorder sought dietary interventions to complement her medication and therapy.
  - ❖ **Intervention:**
- She was advised to follow the Mediterranean diet, with a focus on increasing her intake of fruits, vegetables, whole grains, legumes, nuts, seeds, and olive oil, while reducing her consumption of processed foods and red meat.
  - ❖ **Outcome:**
- After three months, she reported significant improvements in her mood, energy levels, and overall well-being. Her depressive symptoms were reduced, and she experienced fewer mood swings.
  - ❖ **Key Takeaways:**
- The anti-inflammatory and nutrient-rich nature of the Mediterranean diet can significantly improve depressive symptoms and enhance overall mental health.

- o **Case Study 2: Reducing Anxiety with Probiotics and Omega-3 Fatty Acids:**
  - ❖ **Background:**
- A 30-year-old man with generalized anxiety disorder (GAD) sought natural ways to manage his anxiety alongside his prescribed medication.
  - ❖ **Intervention:**
- He was advised to increase his intake of probiotics (through fermented foods and supplements) and omega-3 fatty acids (through fatty fish and fish oil supplements).
  - ❖ **Outcome:**
- After two months, he reported a noticeable reduction in his anxiety levels, better sleep quality, and improved overall mood. He felt more relaxed and less stressed.
  - ❖ **Key Takeaways:**
- Combining probiotics and omega-3 fatty acids can effectively reduce anxiety symptoms by supporting gut health and reducing inflammation.

Conclusion:

Effective management of depression and anxiety can be significantly enhanced through targeted nutritional strategies. Key nutrients like omega-3 fatty acids, B vitamins, magnesium, and vitamin D play crucial roles in mood regulation and brain function. Dietary patterns such as the Mediterranean diet and anti-inflammatory diets offer comprehensive approaches to supporting mental health. By incorporating these dietary strategies, individuals can experience improved mood, reduced anxiety, and overall better mental well-being. The next chapter will delve into the role of nutrition in neurodevelopmental disorders, providing insights and practical guidance for dietary interventions to support children and adults with these conditions.

Chapter 7
The Role of Nutrition in Brain Development and Neurobehavioral Conditions

The developing brain is highly sensitive, what it receives early on can shape not just behavior, but the way a person experiences the world.

I. Autism Spectrum Disorders (ASD):

- **The Role of Nutrition in ASD:**
  - **Gut-Brain Axis:**
    - ❖ **Overview:**
- The gut-brain axis is a bidirectional communication system between the gastrointestinal tract and the brain, influenced by the gut microbiota.
    - ❖ **Impact on ASD:**
- Children with ASD often have gastrointestinal issues, which can exacerbate behavioral and cognitive symptoms. Improving gut health can positively impact symptoms of ASD.

- **Nutritional Strategies:**
  - **Probiotics and Prebiotics:**
    - ❖ **Role:**
- Probiotics (beneficial bacteria) and prebiotics (food for these bacteria) help balance the gut microbiota, reducing gastrointestinal issues and potentially improving ASD symptoms.
    - ❖ **Sources:**
- **Probiotics:** yogurt, kefir, sauerkraut, kimchi.
- **Prebiotics:** garlic, onions, bananas, whole grains.

- o **Gluten-Free, Casein-Free Diet (GFCF):**
  - ❖ **Overview:**
- This diet eliminates gluten (found in wheat, barley, and rye) and casein (found in dairy products).
  - ❖ **Impact on ASD:**
- Some studies suggest that a GFCF diet can reduce symptoms in children with ASD who have sensitivities to these proteins, although results are mixed and more research is needed.
  - ❖ **Practical Tips:**
- Substitute gluten-containing grains with gluten-free alternatives (such as rice, quinoa, and corn) and dairy products with plant-based options (such as almond milk and soy yogurt).

- • **Essential Nutrients:**
  - o **Omega-3 Fatty Acids:**
    - ❖ **Role:**
- Omega-3 fatty acids support brain development and function, and they may reduce inflammation and oxidative stress in the brain.
    - ❖ **Sources:**
- Fatty fish, flaxseeds, chia seeds, walnuts, fish oil supplements.
    - ❖ **Research Evidence:**
- Some studies have found that omega-3 supplementation can improve social interaction and reduce hyperactivity in children with ASD.
  - o **Vitamin D:**
    - ❖ **Role:**
- Vitamin D supports brain function and development, and it may modulate immune responses.
    - ❖ **Sources:**
- Sunlight exposure, fatty fish, fortified dairy products, supplements.

❖ **Research Evidence:**

- Low levels of vitamin D have been observed in children with ASD. Supplementation may help improve symptoms, although more research is needed.

II. <u>ADHD and Diet:</u>

- **The Role of Nutrition in ADHD:**
  - **Elimination Diets:**
    - ❖ **Overview:**

- Elimination diets involve removing specific foods or additives that may trigger symptoms of ADHD and then gradually reintroducing them to identify sensitivities.

    - ❖ **Common Triggers:**

- Artificial colors and flavors, preservatives, sugar, and certain food allergens.

    - ❖ **Research Evidence:**

- Some studies suggest that elimination diets can reduce ADHD symptoms in children sensitive to certain foods or additives.

    - ❖ **Practical Tips:**

- Work with a healthcare professional to design and implement an elimination diet safely and effectively.

- **Essential Nutrients:**
  - **Omega-3 Fatty Acids:**
    - ❖ **Role:**

- Omega-3 fatty acids are crucial for brain health and function. They may reduce hyperactivity and improve attention in children with ADHD.

    - ❖ **Sources:**

- Fatty fish, flaxseeds, chia seeds, walnuts, fish oil supplements.

❖ **Research Evidence:**

- Studies have shown that omega-3 supplementation can improve symptoms of ADHD, particularly in children with low baseline levels.

    o **Iron:**

        ❖ **Role:**

- Iron is essential for oxygen transport and neurotransmitter function. Deficiency can impair cognitive function and increase hyperactivity.

        ❖ **Sources:**

- Red meat, poultry, fish, beans, fortified cereals, spinach.

        ❖ **Research Evidence:**

- Children with ADHD are more likely to have low iron levels. Supplementation may improve symptoms in those with iron deficiency.

    o **Zinc:**

        ❖ **Role:**

- Zinc is involved in neurotransmitter metabolism and immune function. It can influence attention and behavior.

        ❖ **Sources:**

- Meat, shellfish, legumes, seeds, nuts, dairy products.

        ❖ **Research Evidence:**

- Some studies have found that zinc supplementation can reduce hyperactivity and improve attention in children with ADHD, particularly in those with zinc deficiency.

III.　Other Neurodevelopmental Conditions:

- **Role of Diet and Nutrition:**
  - **General Strategies:**
- Emphasize whole foods and balanced diets rich in essential nutrients to support overall brain health and development.
- Avoid processed foods, artificial additives, and potential allergens that may exacerbate symptoms.

- **Nutritional Interventions:**
  - **Phenylketonuria (PKU):**
    - ❖ **Overview:**
- PKU is a genetic disorder that affects the metabolism of the amino acid phenylalanine.
    - ❖ **Dietary Management:**
- Individuals with PKU must follow a low-phenylalanine diet to prevent cognitive impairment and other complications.
- Avoid high-protein foods (such as meat, fish, dairy, nuts, and soy) and use specialized low-phenylalanine products.
  - **Cerebral Palsy (CP):**
    - ❖ **Overview:**
- CP is a group of disorders that affect movement and muscle tone, often accompanied by cognitive and sensory impairments.
    - ❖ **Dietary Considerations:**
- Ensure adequate nutrient intake to support growth and development, considering potential feeding difficulties.
- Work with a healthcare team to address specific nutritional needs and challenges.

  o **Down Syndrome:**
  - ❖ **Overview:**
- Down syndrome is a genetic disorder caused by the presence of an extra chromosome 21.
  - ❖ **Nutritional Strategies:**
- Emphasize a balanced diet to support overall health and development.
- Monitor for specific nutritional deficiencies (such as thyroid function and immune support) and address them as needed.

Conclusion:

Nutritional interventions play a crucial role in managing neurodevelopmental disorders. For conditions like ASD and ADHD, targeted dietary strategies and essential nutrients can significantly improve symptoms and enhance overall well-being. Addressing gut health, eliminating potential dietary triggers, and ensuring adequate intake of key nutrients such as omega-3 fatty acids, vitamins, and minerals are essential components of effective nutritional therapy. By adopting these strategies, individuals with neurodevelopmental disorders can experience improved cognitive function, behavior, and quality of life. The next chapter will present detailed case studies that demonstrate the real-life application of these nutritional interventions, providing valuable insights and practical guidance for clinicians and caregivers.

Chapter 8
Real-Life Transformations:
How Nutrition Changed Mental Health Outcomes

Behind every clinical concept is a real human story, and sometimes, small nutritional changes lead to outcomes no one expected.

I. Individual Cases: Detailed Case Studies Demonstrating the Impact of Nutrition on Mental Health

- **Case Study 1: Overcoming Depression with a Nutrient-Dense Diet**
  - **Background:**
- **Patient:** Sarah, a 35-year-old woman with chronic depression.
- **Symptoms:** Persistent sadness, low energy, difficulty concentrating, disrupted sleep patterns.
- **Previous Treatments:** Antidepressants and psychotherapy with minimal improvement.
  - **Nutritional Assessment:**
- **Dietary Habits:** High intake of processed foods, sugary snacks, caffeinated beverages; low consumption of fruits, vegetables, whole grains.
  - **Intervention:**
- **Dietary Changes:** Transition to a Mediterranean diet rich in fruits, vegetables, whole grains, lean proteins, healthy fats (e.g., fish, nuts, olive oil).
- **Supplementation:** Addition of omega-3 fatty acids, B vitamins, magnesium.

- o **Outcome:**
- **Results:** Significant improvement in mood, energy levels, concentration, and sleep within three months. Reduction in depressive symptoms and reliance on medication.

- **Case Study 2: Reducing Anxiety Through Gut Health:**
  - o **Background:**
- **Patient:** John, a 28-year-old man with severe anxiety and occasional panic attacks.
- **Symptoms:** Persistent worry, restlessness, muscle tension, gastrointestinal issues.
- **Previous Treatments:** Anti-anxiety medications, cognitive-behavioral therapy with limited success.
  - o **Nutritional Assessment:**
- **Dietary Habits:** High intake of processed foods, artificial sweeteners, low fiber.
  - o **Intervention:**
- **Dietary Changes:** Introduction of a diet rich in prebiotic and probiotic foods (e.g., yogurt, sauerkraut), high-fiber vegetables, whole grains.
- **Supplementation:** Probiotic supplements, increased intake of magnesium-rich foods.
  - o **Outcome:**
- **Results:** Noticeable reduction in anxiety symptoms and panic attacks within two months. Improved gut health, better digestion, overall well-being.

- **Case Study 3: Managing ADHD with a Balanced Diet:**
  - **Background:**
- **Patient:** Emily, a 10-year-old girl with attention deficit hyperactivity disorder (ADHD).
- **Symptoms:** Hyperactivity, impulsivity, difficulty focusing, behavioral issues.
- **Previous Treatments:** Stimulant medications, behavioral therapy with partial improvement.
  - **Nutritional Assessment:**
- **Dietary Habits:** High consumption of sugary snacks, processed foods, low nutrient density meals.

  - **Intervention:**
- **Dietary Changes:** Incorporation of a balanced diet emphasizing lean proteins, complex carbohydrates, healthy fats, variety of fruits and vegetables. Reduction in sugar, processed food intake.
- **Supplementation:** Omega-3 fatty acids, multivitamin supplement.
  - **Outcome:**
- **Results:** Significant improvement in focus, behavior, academic performance within four months. Reduced hyperactivity, better overall health.

II. <u>Lessons Learned: Key Takeaways from Each Case</u>

- **Nutrient-Dense Diets Can Significantly Alleviate Depressive Symptoms:**
- Transitioning to a diet rich in whole foods, such as the Mediterranean diet, significantly alleviates depressive symptoms by providing essential nutrients that support brain health.

- **Omega-3 Fatty Acids, B Vitamins, and Magnesium Play Critical Roles in Mental Health:**
- **Omega-3 Fatty Acids:** Crucial for brain cell membrane structure and function, anti-inflammatory properties. Found in fatty fish, flaxseeds, walnuts.
- **B Vitamins:** Essential for neurotransmitter synthesis (e.g., serotonin, dopamine). Found in leafy greens, whole grains, eggs.
- **Magnesium:** Involved in over 300 biochemical reactions, regulates nervous system, reduces anxiety and depression. Found in leafy greens, nuts, seeds.

- **Consistency and Adherence to Dietary Changes are Crucial for Long-Term Benefits**
- Long-term mental health improvements require consistent adherence to dietary changes.

  - **Strategies:**
- **Regular Follow-Ups:** Maintain accountability, address challenges.
- **Support Systems:** Involve family, join support groups.
- **Education and Empowerment:** Educate patients on diet-mental health link, provide practical guidance.
- **Flexibility and Personalization:** Tailor diet plans to individual preferences, lifestyles.

III. <u>Practical Tips for Clinicians: How to Apply These Lessons in Clinical Practice:</u>

- **Regular Monitoring:**
- Conduct regular nutritional assessments, follow-ups to ensure adherence, make necessary adjustments.

- **Collaborative Approach:**
- Work with dietitians, nutritionists to develop comprehensive dietary plans tailored to individual needs.

- **Patient Education:**
- Educate patients on importance of nutrition in mental health, provide practical guidance on making sustainable dietary changes.

- **Support Systems:**
- Encourage involvement of family members, support groups to foster a supportive environment for dietary changes.

<u>Conclusion:</u>

These case studies highlight the transformative potential of nutritional interventions in mental health care. By integrating personalized dietary strategies into treatment plans, clinicians can help patients achieve significant and lasting improvements in their mental well-being. Nutrient-dense diets, targeted supplementation, and consistent adherence to dietary changes are crucial for optimizing mental health. Through a collaborative and patient-centered approach, nutrition can become a powerful tool in the holistic management of mental health conditions.

Chapter 9
Bringing Nutrition into Mental Health Care:
Practical Clinical Applications

Knowing the science is one thing, but applying it in real-life situations is where true impact begins.

I. Assessment and Diagnosis:

- **Comprehensive Nutritional Assessment:**
  - **Initial Consultation:**
- Conduct a thorough evaluation of the patient's dietary habits, including a detailed food diary covering at least one week.
- Assess lifestyle factors such as sleep patterns, physical activity, and stress levels that may influence nutritional status.
- Review medical history, including any existing conditions, medications, and supplements.
  - **Nutrient Deficiency Screening:**
- Identify common nutrient deficiencies that may impact mental health, such as omega-3 fatty acids, vitamins (B12, D, C), and minerals (magnesium, zinc, iron).
- Utilize blood tests and other diagnostic tools to confirm deficiencies and establish baseline levels for monitoring progress.

- **Psychological and Behavioral Assessment:**
- Evaluate the patient's mental health status using standardized tools and clinical interviews.
- Identify any disordered eating patterns, food aversions, or psychological barriers to healthy eating.

II. Developing Nutritional Plans:

- **Personalized Dietary Interventions:**
  - **Goal Setting:**
- Collaborate with the patient to set realistic and achievable dietary goals that align with their mental health needs and lifestyle.
- Prioritize gradual changes to foster sustainable habits and avoid overwhelming the patient.

- **Customized Meal Plans:**
- Create individualized meal plans that emphasize whole foods, balance macronutrients, and include a variety of nutrient-dense options.
- Address specific dietary restrictions, preferences, and cultural considerations to enhance adherence.

- **Supplement Recommendations:**
- Determine the need for supplements based on identified nutrient deficiencies and dietary gaps.
- Provide guidance on appropriate dosages, reputable brands, and potential interactions with medications.

III. Implementing and Monitoring Dietary Interventions:

- **Patient Education and Empowerment:**
  - **Nutritional Counseling:**
- Offer educational sessions to help patients understand the connection between nutrition and mental health.
- Provide practical tips for meal planning, grocery shopping, and cooking to empower patients to make healthier choices.

  o **Behavioral Strategies:**
- Incorporate behavioral techniques such as mindful eating, portion control, and stress management to support dietary changes.
- Address emotional eating and develop coping mechanisms for managing cravings and triggers.

  • **Regular Monitoring and Follow-Up:**
  o **Progress Tracking:**
- Schedule regular follow-up appointments to monitor the patient's progress, assess compliance, and address any challenges.
- Utilize tools such as food diaries, symptom trackers, and biometric measurements to gather data and adjust interventions as needed.
  o **Outcome Evaluation:**
- Evaluate the impact of dietary changes on mental health symptoms, cognitive function, and overall well-being.
- Adjust nutritional plans based on patient feedback and clinical observations to optimize outcomes.

IV. <u>Collaboration with Dietitians and Nutritionists:</u>

  • **Multidisciplinary Approach:**
  o **Integrated Care Team:**
- Form collaborative partnerships with dietitians, nutritionists, and other healthcare professionals to provide comprehensive care.
- Ensure clear communication and coordination between team members to align treatment goals and interventions.
  o **Referral Systems:**
- Establish referral pathways to connect patients with specialized nutritional support when needed.

- Facilitate access to resources such as cooking classes, support groups, and community programs that promote healthy eating.

V.   <u>Addressing Challenges and Barriers:</u>

- **Common Obstacles:**
  - **Financial Constraints:**
- Recognize the financial barriers that may limit access to healthy foods and supplements.
- Provide resources and strategies for affordable healthy eating, such as budget-friendly recipes and tips for shopping on a budget.

  - **Psychological Resistance:**
- Identify and address psychological resistance to dietary changes, including fear of change, lack of motivation, and low self-efficacy.
- Utilize motivational interviewing and other therapeutic techniques to foster a positive attitude towards nutrition.

- **Cultural Sensitivity:**
  - **Respecting Cultural Practices:**
- Respect and incorporate cultural dietary practices and preferences into nutritional plans.
- Work with patients to find culturally appropriate and nutritionally balanced options that align with their traditions and values.

  - **Language and Communication:**
- Provide educational materials and counseling in the patient's preferred language to enhance understanding and engagement.

- Use culturally relevant examples and analogies to explain nutritional concepts.

Conclusion:

Integrating nutrition into mental health care requires a holistic and patient-centered approach. By conducting comprehensive assessments, developing personalized dietary interventions, and collaborating with a multidisciplinary team, clinicians can effectively address the nutritional needs of their patients. Overcoming challenges such as financial constraints and psychological resistance is crucial to fostering sustainable dietary changes and improving mental health outcomes. The next chapter will explore the scientific debates, practical challenges, and future directions in nutritional psychiatry, providing a broader context for ongoing research and innovation in this field.

Chapter 10
The Controversies, Limitations,
and Truths Behind Nutritional Psychiatry

Not everything in nutritional psychiatry is clear-cut, and understanding the uncertainty is just as important as understanding the science.

Nutritional psychiatry, a burgeoning field, investigates the impact of diet on mental health. Despite promising findings, integrating nutrition into psychiatric care faces various challenges and controversies. This chapter provides an in-depth examination of these issues, highlighting both the complexities and the potential benefits of this interdisciplinary approach.

I. <u>Scientific Debates:</u>

- **Causality vs. Correlation:**

One of the core debates in nutritional psychiatry centers around the distinction between causality and correlation. While numerous studies suggest a strong correlation between diet and mental health, proving direct causation remains challenging. Observational studies, which form the bulk of current research, can demonstrate associations but not definitive causal relationships. Critics argue that other variables, such as lifestyle factors or pre-existing health conditions, might influence these findings. Randomized controlled trials (RCTs) are needed to establish causation, but they are complex and costly to conduct in this field.

- **Effectiveness of Dietary Interventions:**

The effectiveness of dietary interventions compared to conventional psychiatric treatments is another contentious topic. Some researchers and clinicians believe that while nutrition plays a supportive role, it cannot replace established treatments such as medication and psychotherapy. However, proponents of nutritional psychiatry argue that diet should be considered an integral part of a comprehensive treatment plan, potentially enhancing the effectiveness of conventional therapies and improving overall patient outcomes.

- **Nutritional Supplements:**

The use of nutritional supplements in mental health care is a subject of ongoing debate. While some studies indicate that certain supplements, such as omega-3 fatty acids, B vitamins, and probiotics, can have beneficial effects on mental health, others question their efficacy and safety. Concerns about the regulation and quality control of supplements also contribute to this debate, highlighting the need for more rigorous research and standardized guidelines.

II. <u>Practical Challenges:</u>

- **Lack of Standardized Guidelines:**

One of the major practical challenges in nutritional psychiatry is the lack of standardized guidelines. Unlike other areas of medicine, nutritional psychiatry does not yet have universally accepted protocols. This lack of standardization can lead to variability in care and uncertainty about the best practices. Developing evidence-based guidelines and integrating them into clinical practice is crucial for the field's advancement.

- **Patient Compliance:**

Changing dietary habits can be particularly challenging for individuals with mental health issues. Conditions like depression and anxiety can affect motivation, energy levels, and cognitive function, making it difficult for patients to adhere to new dietary regimes. Moreover, socioeconomic factors, such as access to healthy food, financial constraints, and cultural preferences, can further complicate adherence to nutritional recommendations. Clinicians must consider these factors when designing and implementing dietary interventions.

- **Training and Education:**

There is a need for enhanced training and education for healthcare professionals in nutritional psychiatry. Many clinicians lack sufficient knowledge about the role of nutrition in mental health and are not adequately equipped to provide dietary advice or interventions. Integrating nutrition education into medical and psychiatric training programs can help bridge this gap and promote a more holistic approach to mental health care.

III. <u>Future Directions:</u>

• Personalized Nutrition:

Personalized nutrition, which tailors dietary recommendations to an individual's genetic profile, lifestyle, and health status, represents a promising future direction for nutritional psychiatry. Advances in genomics and metabolomics are paving the way for more precise and effective dietary interventions. Personalized nutrition could address individual variations in dietary response, making interventions more effective and reducing the risk of adverse effects.

• Innovative Therapies:

The development of innovative nutritional therapies, such as functional foods and targeted supplements, holds significant potential. Functional foods are specifically designed to have health benefits beyond basic nutrition, and targeted supplements can provide specific nutrients that may be deficient in individuals with mental health conditions. These therapies, developed through rigorous scientific research, could offer new avenues for treatment and support mental health more effectively.

• Multidisciplinary Collaboration:

Collaborative efforts between nutritionists, psychiatrists, psychologists, and other healthcare professionals are essential for advancing nutritional psychiatry. A multidisciplinary approach ensures that patients receive comprehensive care that addresses both their physical and mental health needs. By fostering collaboration and communication among healthcare providers, the field can move towards more integrative and holistic treatment models.

Conclusion:

Nutritional psychiatry, despite its challenges and controversies, holds significant promise for enhancing mental health care. While scientific debates and practical obstacles remain, ongoing research, personalized approaches, and collaborative efforts are paving the way for a more integrated understanding of the relationship between diet and mental health. By navigating these complexities and embracing the potential of nutritional interventions, both clinicians and patients can benefit from a more holistic approach to mental health.

As readers continue through this book, they will gain deeper insights into the intricacies of nutritional psychiatry. Understanding the challenges and engaging with the controversies will equip them to navigate this evolving landscape with greater confidence and optimism, ultimately contributing to better mental health outcomes.

Chapter 11
Where Science Is Headed:
The Future of Nutrition and Mental Health

The field is evolving fast, and what we understand today may only be the beginning of a much deeper connection.

As the field of nutritional psychiatry continues to evolve, it opens up numerous possibilities for research and innovation. This chapter delves into the future directions that could shape the landscape of mental health care, highlighting cutting-edge research, innovative therapies, and emerging trends that promise to deepen our understanding of the intricate link between nutrition and mental health.

I. **Cutting-Edge Research:**

- **Epigenetics and Nutrition:**

One of the most exciting areas of research in nutritional psychiatry is the study of epigenetics, which examines how gene expression is influenced by environmental factors, including diet. Epigenetic modifications can affect how genes related to mental health are expressed, potentially leading to new insights into how nutritional interventions can modify the risk and progression of mental health disorders. For instance, research is exploring how specific nutrients like folate, vitamin B12, and omega-3 fatty acids can influence epigenetic mechanisms and impact mental health.

- **Microbiome and Mental Health:**

The gut-brain axis and the role of the microbiome in mental health are gaining significant attention. Future research aims to further elucidate how gut bacteria influence brain function and behavior. Studies are investigating the potential of prebiotics, probiotics, and synbiotics to modulate the microbiome and improve mental health outcomes. Advanced techniques like metagenomics and metabolomics are being used to identify specific microbial strains and metabolic pathways that contribute to mental health, paving the way for targeted microbiome-based therapies.

- **Nutritional Neuroscience:**

Nutritional neuroscience focuses on understanding how nutrients affect brain function and structure. Future research in this field aims to identify the precise mechanisms by which different nutrients influence neural pathways, neurotransmitter systems, and neuroplasticity. For example, the impact of antioxidants, polyphenols, and other bioactive compounds on reducing oxidative stress and inflammation in the brain is a key area of interest. These insights could lead to the development of novel nutritional interventions that support cognitive health and prevent neurodegenerative diseases.

II. <u>**Innovative Therapies:**</u>

- **Functional Foods:**

Functional foods, which contain bioactive compounds with health benefits beyond basic nutrition, represent a promising area of innovation. Future developments may include foods specifically formulated to enhance mental health, such as beverages enriched with adaptogens to reduce stress, snacks fortified with omega-3 fatty acids to support cognitive function, or meals designed to balance blood sugar levels and improve mood stability. The integration of functional foods into daily diets could offer a convenient and effective way to support mental well-being.

- **Personalized Nutrition:**

Advances in genetic testing and precision medicine are paving the way for personalized nutrition. By analyzing an individual's genetic profile, microbiome composition, and metabolic markers, personalized dietary plans can be developed to optimize mental health. This approach acknowledges that each person responds differently to nutrients based on their unique biological makeup. Personalized nutrition aims to tailor interventions that address specific deficiencies, intolerances, and metabolic variations, enhancing the efficacy of dietary strategies in managing mental health conditions.

- **Digital Health Technologies:**

The integration of digital health technologies into nutritional psychiatry is transforming how dietary interventions are delivered and monitored. Mobile apps, wearable devices, and telehealth platforms are being developed to track dietary intake, monitor mental health symptoms, and provide personalized recommendations in real-time. These technologies can enhance patient engagement, improve adherence to dietary plans, and facilitate remote support from healthcare providers. Future innovations may include AI-driven platforms that analyze data from multiple sources to offer dynamic and adaptive nutritional guidance.

III. <u>Research Opportunities:</u>

- ### Longitudinal Studies:

There is a growing need for long-term, longitudinal studies to better understand the sustained effects of nutritional interventions on mental health. These studies can provide valuable insights into how dietary changes impact mental health over extended periods, identify potential long-term benefits and risks, and inform guidelines for maintenance and prevention strategies. Longitudinal research can also help clarify the temporal relationship between diet and mental health outcomes, contributing to a more nuanced understanding of causality.

- ### Integrative Approaches:

Exploring integrative approaches that combine nutrition with other therapies offers a rich area for future research. For example, studying the synergistic effects of combining dietary interventions with mindfulness practices, exercise, or pharmacotherapy could reveal new strategies for enhancing mental health. Integrative approaches recognize the multifaceted nature of mental health and aim to address it from multiple angles, potentially leading to more comprehensive and effective treatment protocols.

- ### Socioeconomic and Cultural Factors:

Understanding the impact of socioeconomic and cultural factors on the implementation and effectiveness of nutritional interventions is crucial for developing inclusive and accessible strategies. Future research should examine how factors such as income, education, food availability, and cultural dietary practices influence the adoption and success of nutritional psychiatry. This knowledge can guide the creation of tailored interventions that are culturally sensitive and equitable, ensuring that the benefits of nutritional psychiatry reach diverse populations.

Conclusion:

The future of nutritional psychiatry is filled with potential and promise. As research continues to uncover the complex interactions between diet and mental health, innovative therapies and personalized approaches are emerging to revolutionize mental health care. By embracing cutting-edge research, leveraging digital health technologies, and adopting integrative and inclusive strategies, the field is poised to make significant strides in improving mental health outcomes.

As readers progress through this book, they will gain a deeper appreciation for the exciting developments and opportunities in nutritional psychiatry. Understanding these future directions will empower clinicians and patients alike to embrace the evolving landscape of mental health care, fostering a more holistic and effective approach to well-being.

Chapter 12
Tools, Resources, and Practical Support for Real-World Application

Information alone does not create change, what matters is how you use it in everyday life.

As the field of nutritional psychiatry continues to grow, having access to the right resources and tools is crucial for both clinicians and patients. This chapter aims to provide a comprehensive guide to various resources that can support the implementation of nutritional interventions in mental health care. From supplement guides to practical recipes, these tools are designed to enhance understanding and application of nutritional psychiatry principles.

I. <u>Supplement Guides:</u>

• Vitamins and Minerals:

Understanding the role of vitamins and minerals in mental health is essential for effective dietary planning. This section offers detailed guides on key nutrients, their benefits, recommended daily allowances, and potential sources:

- **Vitamin B Complex:** Crucial for brain function and energy production. Found in whole grains, meat, eggs, and dairy products.
- **Vitamin D:** Supports mood regulation and cognitive function. Obtained from sunlight exposure, fatty fish, and fortified foods.
- **Vitamin C:** Important for neurotransmitter synthesis and antioxidant protection. Found in fruits like oranges, strawberries, and kiwi.

- **Magnesium:** Aids in relaxation and stress reduction. Present in nuts, seeds, leafy greens, and whole grains.
- **Zinc:** Essential for neuroplasticity and immune function. Found in meat, shellfish, legumes, and seeds.
- **Iron:** Vital for oxygen transport and cognitive development. Sourced from red meat, beans, lentils, and fortified cereals.

- **Herbal Supplements:**

Herbal supplements can offer additional support for mental health. This section provides an overview of commonly used herbs, their effects, and guidelines for use:

- **St. John's Wort:** Known for its antidepressant properties. Caution advised due to potential interactions with medications.
- **Valerian Root:** Used for anxiety and sleep disorders. Typically taken as a tea or supplement.
- **Ashwagandha:** An adaptogen that helps manage stress and anxiety. Available in powder or capsule form.
- **Rhodiola Rosea:** Enhances resilience to stress and fatigue. Commonly found in capsule or extract form.

II. Recipes for Mental Wellness:

Nutritious and easy-to-prepare recipes can make it easier for patients to adopt dietary changes. This section includes a variety of recipes designed to support mental health:

- **Breakfast:**
- **Berry and Nut Overnight Oats:** A combination of oats, almond milk, mixed berries, chia seeds, and nuts soaked overnight.

- **Spinach and Feta Omelette:** Made with fresh spinach, feta cheese, eggs, and a dash of olive oil.

- **Lunch:**
- **Quinoa and Black Bean Salad:** A mix of cooked quinoa, black beans, corn, bell peppers, avocado, and a lime-cilantro dressing.
- **Salmon and Avocado Wrap:** Whole-grain wrap filled with grilled salmon, avocado, spinach, and a yogurt-based dressing.

- **Dinner:**
- **Mediterranean Chickpea Stew:** A hearty stew with chickpeas, tomatoes, spinach, onions, garlic, and a blend of Mediterranean spices.
- **Grilled Chicken with Sweet Potato Mash:** Grilled chicken breast served with mashed sweet potatoes and steamed broccoli.

- **Snacks:**
- **Trail Mix:** A blend of nuts, seeds, dried fruit, and dark chocolate chunks.
- **Greek Yogurt with Honey and Walnuts:** Greek yogurt topped with a drizzle of honey and a handful of walnuts.

III. <u>Additional Resources:</u>

- ### Books and Journals:

Staying informed about the latest research and developments in nutritional psychiatry is essential. This section lists key books and academic journals:

- o **Books:**
- - "The Good Mood Diet" by Susan Kleiner.
- - "The Anti-Anxiety Food Solution" by Trudy Scott.
- - "Nutritional Psychiatry" by Ted Dinan and John F. Cryan.

- o **Journals:**
- - Journal of Nutritional Biochemistry.
- - Nutrition Reviews.
- - The American Journal of Clinical Nutrition.

- o **Websites and Online Platforms:**

Reliable online resources can provide additional information and support. Here are some recommended websites and platforms:

- **Mental Health Foundation:** Provides information on the link between nutrition and mental health.
- **Mind:** Offers resources and support for mental health, including dietary advice.
- **Nutritional Psychiatry Network:** A platform for professionals to share research and insights.
- **Healthline:** Features articles and guides on nutrition and mental health.

- **Tools for Clinicians:**
  - **Assessment Tools:**

  Effective assessment is key to integrating nutrition into mental health care. This section provides tools and questionnaires for evaluating nutritional status:

  - **Nutritional Assessment Questionnaire:** A comprehensive tool to assess dietary habits, nutrient intake, and potential deficiencies.
  - **Food Frequency Questionnaire (FFQ):** Helps track the frequency and variety of food intake over a specific period.
  - **Dietary Recall:** A method to record and analyze a patient's dietary intake over the past 24 hours.

  - **Treatment Planning:**

  Developing tailored nutritional plans is essential for patient success. This section offers guidelines for creating effective treatment plans:

  - **Individualized Nutrition Plans:** Steps for creating personalized dietary recommendations based on assessment findings.
  - **Goal Setting:** Techniques for setting realistic and achievable dietary goals with patients.
  - **Monitoring Progress:** Tools for tracking patient progress and adjusting plans as needed.

  - **Collaboration with Nutritionists:**

  Working with nutritionists can enhance the quality of care. This section emphasizes the importance of multidisciplinary collaboration:

  - **Referral Process:** Guidelines for referring patients to nutritionists and dietitians.
  - **Collaborative Care Models:** Examples of integrated care approaches that combine psychiatric and nutritional expertise.

- **Communication Strategies:** Tips for effective communication and coordination between mental health professionals and nutritionists.

<u>Conclusion:</u>

Having the right resources and tools is essential for implementing nutritional interventions in mental health care effectively. By utilizing supplement guides, nutritious recipes, reliable additional resources, and practical tools for clinicians, both patients and healthcare providers can benefit from a more holistic approach to mental health. As the field of nutritional psychiatry continues to evolve, staying informed and equipped with the best resources will be key to improving mental health outcomes.

This chapter aims to empower readers with the knowledge and tools they need to incorporate nutrition into their mental health practices, fostering a more integrative and effective approach to mental well-being.

Chapter 13
Hydration and the Brain:
The Overlooked Factor in Mental Clarity

Before searching for complex explanations, consider this: even mild dehydration can quietly affect how clearly you think and feel.

Hydration is a fundamental yet often overlooked aspect of maintaining optimal mental health. Water is essential for a variety of bodily functions, including those of the brain. Even mild dehydration can negatively impact mood, cognitive abilities, and overall mental well-being. This chapter delves deeply into the importance of water for brain function, the effects of dehydration on cognitive and emotional health, and practical strategies for maintaining optimal hydration to support mental health.

I.   **The Importance of Water for Brain Function:**

Water is crucial for numerous physiological processes that keep the brain functioning optimally. The brain is composed of approximately 75% water, and this high-water content is essential for:

- **Neurotransmitter Synthesis:**

Neurotransmitters are chemical messengers that transmit signals between nerve cells. Proper hydration supports the synthesis and function of neurotransmitters, which are critical for mood regulation and cognitive functions such as learning, memory, and concentration. Dehydration can disrupt the balance of neurotransmitters, potentially leading to mood disorders and cognitive impairments.

• Nutrient Transport:

Water facilitates the transport of nutrients to brain cells. Essential nutrients like glucose, amino acids, and vitamins rely on water for their absorption and distribution throughout the brain. Adequate hydration ensures that brain cells receive the nutrients they need to function effectively, supporting overall cognitive health and mental performance.

• Toxin Removal:

Hydration is vital for the removal of metabolic waste products and toxins from the brain. The brain's detoxification processes depend on an adequate supply of water to flush out harmful substances that can accumulate and impair cognitive functions. Chronic dehydration can lead to the build-up of toxins, contributing to cognitive decline and mental fatigue.

• Temperature Regulation:

Water helps maintain the brain's optimal temperature. The brain is highly sensitive to temperature changes, and even slight variations can affect cognitive functions. Hydration supports the brain's ability to regulate its temperature, ensuring that neural processes operate efficiently and preventing heat-related cognitive impairments.

II.   <u>Dehydration and Cognitive Impairment:</u>

Even mild dehydration can have significant negative effects on cognitive performance and emotional health. The brain requires a consistent supply of water to function properly, and dehydration can disrupt this balance, leading to:

- **Impaired Cognitive Function:**

Dehydration can impair various aspects of cognitive function, including short-term memory, attention, and executive function. Studies have shown that even a 1-2% reduction in body water can negatively affect cognitive tasks that require focus, attention, and complex thinking. Students, professionals, and individuals performing mentally demanding tasks are particularly susceptible to these impairments.

- **Mood Disturbances:**

Hydration levels are closely linked to mood regulation. Dehydration has been associated with increased feelings of anxiety, irritability, and depression. These mood disturbances can arise due to the brain's sensitivity to water balance and its impact on neurotransmitter function. Additionally, dehydration can lead to fatigue, further exacerbating negative mood states and reducing overall quality of life.

- **Reduced Alertness and Focus:**

Lack of adequate hydration can lead to reduced alertness and a general sense of mental fatigue. Individuals may experience difficulty staying focused, maintaining attention, and processing information quickly. This reduction in cognitive sharpness can affect daily activities, work performance, and overall productivity.

- **Increased Stress Response:**

Dehydration can increase the body's stress response, leading to elevated levels of cortisol, the stress hormone. High cortisol levels can negatively impact both physical and mental health, contributing to feelings of stress, anxiety, and tension. Chronic dehydration can perpetuate this stress response, creating a cycle of heightened stress and poor hydration.

III.   Optimal Hydration Strategies:

Maintaining optimal hydration is essential for supporting mental health. Implementing effective hydration strategies can help ensure that the brain functions at its best:

- **Regular Water Intake:**

Aim to drink at least 8-10 glasses of water daily, with adjustments based on individual needs, activity levels, and environmental conditions. Establishing a routine for regular water consumption throughout the day can help maintain consistent hydration levels. Consider carrying a reusable water bottle and setting reminders to drink water, especially during busy or stressful periods.

- **Incorporate Hydrating Foods:**

Include water-rich foods in your diet to supplement your water intake. Fruits like watermelon, oranges, and strawberries, as well as vegetables like cucumbers, lettuce, and zucchini, have high water content and provide additional hydration. Soups, smoothies, and herbal teas are also excellent options for increasing fluid intake while enjoying nutritious and delicious meals.

- **Monitor Hydration Levels:**

Pay attention to signs of dehydration, such as dry mouth, dark urine, and decreased urine output. Monitoring these indicators can help you stay aware of your hydration status and make timely adjustments. Using hydration apps or setting reminders on your phone can support regular water intake and prevent unintentional dehydration.

- **Hydrate Before, During, and After Exercise:**

Physical activity increases water loss through sweat, making it essential to hydrate adequately before, during, and after exercise. Pre-hydration ensures that your body starts with sufficient water levels, while drinking water during exercise helps maintain performance and prevent dehydration. Post-exercise hydration is crucial for replenishing lost fluids and supporting recovery. Sports drinks with electrolytes can be beneficial for intense or prolonged exercise, as they help restore electrolyte balance.

- **Limit Diuretics:**

Be mindful of the intake of diuretics such as caffeine and alcohol, which can increase water loss. While moderate consumption of these beverages is generally acceptable, excessive intake can lead to dehydration. Balance the consumption of diuretics with adequate water intake to maintain optimal hydration levels. Consider choosing herbal teas or decaffeinated beverages as alternatives to reduce diuretic effects.

- **Create Hydration Habits:**

Establishing hydration habits can make it easier to maintain adequate water intake. Drink a glass of water upon waking to start the day hydrated, and make it a habit to drink water before and during meals. Setting specific times for water breaks, such as mid-morning and mid-afternoon, can help ensure regular hydration throughout the day. Additionally, keeping water accessible in your home, workplace, and car can encourage frequent consumption.

Conclusion:

Water is fundamental to brain function and overall mental health. Understanding the impact of hydration on cognitive abilities and mood is crucial for promoting mental well-being. By adopting effective hydration strategies, individuals can enhance their cognitive function, improve mood, and support their mental health.

This chapter emphasizes the importance of hydration and provides practical tips for maintaining optimal hydration levels. By integrating these strategies into daily routines, readers can take a proactive approach to their mental well-being, ensuring that their brain and body are adequately hydrated to function at their best. As awareness of the connection between hydration and mental health grows, both individuals and healthcare providers can prioritize water intake as a key component of comprehensive mental health care.

Chapter 14
The Powerful Synergy Between Nutrition, Exercise, and Mental Performance

Your body and mind are not separate systems, and when they work together, the results can be far greater than either alone.

Combining exercise and nutrition offers a powerful approach to enhancing mental health. Both elements independently contribute to brain health and emotional well-being, and their synergistic effects can significantly improve mental performance and mood. This chapter delves into the combined impact of diet and exercise, the role of exercise-induced neurotransmitters, and nutritional strategies to support physical and mental performance.

I.   <u>Synergistic Effects of Diet and Exercise:</u>

The relationship between exercise and nutrition is deeply intertwined, each amplifying the benefits of the other. A balanced diet provides the necessary fuel and nutrients to support physical activity, while regular exercise enhances the body's ability to utilize these nutrients efficiently. Together, they contribute to:

- **Improved Cognitive Function:**

Exercise increases blood flow to the brain, promoting the delivery of oxygen and nutrients essential for cognitive processes. A nutrient-rich diet supports brain health by providing antioxidants, vitamins, and minerals that protect brain cells and improve cognitive function. This combination can lead to enhanced memory, attention, and executive function.

• Enhanced Mood and Emotional Well-Being:

Physical activity stimulates the production of endorphins and other neurotransmitters that promote feelings of happiness and reduce symptoms of depression and anxiety. Nutrition plays a critical role in regulating neurotransmitter levels, with specific nutrients such as omega-3 fatty acids, B vitamins, and amino acids supporting the synthesis and function of mood-regulating chemicals. The combined effects of exercise and a healthy diet can lead to improved emotional stability and overall well-being.

• Increased Energy Levels:

Exercise boosts energy levels by enhancing mitochondrial function and increasing the efficiency of energy production in cells. A balanced diet provides the necessary macronutrients (carbohydrates, proteins, and fats) and micronutrients (vitamins and minerals) to sustain energy levels throughout the day. Together, they help maintain consistent energy, reduce fatigue, and support active lifestyles.

• Stress Reduction:

Both exercise and nutrition play significant roles in stress management. Physical activity helps reduce stress by lowering cortisol levels and promoting relaxation. Nutritional strategies that include foods rich in magnesium, vitamin C, and complex carbohydrates can further support the body's stress response. The synergistic effects of exercise and a balanced diet can lead to better stress management and improved resilience to life's challenges.

II. **Exercise-Induced Neurotransmitters:**

Exercise has a profound impact on the production and regulation of neurotransmitters, which are critical for mental health. Key neurotransmitters influenced by physical activity include:

- **Endorphins:**

Endorphins, often referred to as "feel-good" hormones, are released during exercise and act as natural painkillers and mood enhancers. They contribute to the "runner's high" and help alleviate symptoms of depression and anxiety.

- **Serotonin:**

Exercise increases the availability of tryptophan, an amino acid precursor to serotonin, which plays a crucial role in mood regulation. Higher levels of serotonin are associated with improved mood, reduced anxiety, and better sleep.

- **Dopamine:**

Physical activity stimulates the release of dopamine, a neurotransmitter involved in reward, motivation, and pleasure. Increased dopamine levels can enhance focus, motivation, and feelings of well-being.

- **Norepinephrine:**

Exercise boosts the production of norepinephrine, a neurotransmitter that helps regulate attention, arousal, and the body's response to stress. Higher levels of norepinephrine can improve concentration and reduce symptoms of ADHD.

III. <u>Nutrition to Support Exercise:</u>

Proper nutrition is essential for maximizing the benefits of exercise and supporting overall mental health. Nutritional strategies to enhance physical and mental performance include:

- **Pre-Exercise Nutrition:**

Consuming a balanced meal or snack before exercise provides the necessary energy and nutrients to fuel physical activity. Carbohydrates are the primary energy source, while proteins support muscle repair and growth. Healthy fats can provide sustained energy for longer workouts. Examples of pre-exercise snacks include a banana with almond butter, a yogurt with berries, or a whole-grain toast with avocado.

- **Post-Exercise Nutrition:**

Refueling after exercise is crucial for recovery and muscle repair. A combination of proteins and carbohydrates helps replenish glycogen stores and promote muscle synthesis. Including antioxidants in post-exercise meals can help reduce inflammation and oxidative stress. Examples of post-exercise meals include a protein smoothie with spinach and berries, a chicken and quinoa salad, or a tofu stir-fry with vegetables.

- **Hydration:**

Staying hydrated is essential for optimal exercise performance and recovery. Water is vital for maintaining blood volume, regulating body temperature, and transporting nutrients to muscles. During prolonged or intense exercise, electrolyte-rich drinks can help replenish lost minerals and prevent dehydration.

- **Supplements:**

Certain supplements can support exercise performance and recovery. Protein powders, branched-chain amino acids (BCAAs), and creatine can enhance muscle growth and repair. Omega-3 fatty acids, magnesium, and vitamin D can support overall health and reduce inflammation. It's essential to consult with a healthcare provider before starting any supplement regimen.

Conclusion:

The combined impact of exercise and nutrition offers a powerful approach to enhancing mental health. By understanding the synergistic effects of diet and physical activity, individuals can optimize their mental performance, improve mood, and support overall well-being.

This chapter highlights the importance of integrating regular exercise and a balanced diet into daily routines. By adopting these strategies, readers can take a proactive approach to their mental and physical health, ensuring that they harness the full benefits of both exercise and nutrition. As awareness of the connection between physical activity, nutrition, and mental health grows, individuals can make informed choices that lead to healthier, happier lives.

Chapter 15
Special Diets and Their Real Impact
on Mental Health

Some dietary approaches promise clarity and focus, but the real question is: **what actually works, and for whom?**

Understanding the relationship between diet and mental health is crucial in our ongoing pursuit of well-being. Certain diets have gained prominence for their potential to influence mental clarity, emotional stability, and overall brain function. This chapter delves into the ketogenic diet, intermittent fasting, and gluten-free diets, examining their mechanisms, benefits, challenges, and practical applications in the context of mental health.

I. The Ketogenic Diet and Mental Clarity:

The ketogenic diet is a high-fat, low-carbohydrate diet designed to shift the body into a state of ketosis, where it burns fat for fuel instead of glucose. This shift has significant implications for brain function and mental clarity.

- **Mechanisms of Action:**
- **Ketones as Brain Fuel:** In ketosis, the brain uses ketones instead of glucose for energy, which can provide a more stable and efficient energy source, reducing cognitive fatigue and enhancing mental clarity.
- **Neuroprotection:** The ketogenic diet has been shown to reduce oxidative stress and inflammation, protecting brain cells from damage and potentially mitigating the risk of neurodegenerative diseases.

- **Neurotransmitter Balance:** This diet may increase levels of GABA, a neurotransmitter that calms the nervous system, leading to reduced anxiety and improved mental stability.

- **Mental Health Benefits:**
- **Enhanced Focus:** Many individuals on a ketogenic diet report sharper focus and sustained attention, attributed to the steady supply of ketones as an energy source.
- **Mood Stabilization:** The diet's influence on neurotransmitter levels and inflammation may help stabilize mood, particularly in conditions like bipolar disorder.
- **Depression Management:** Emerging research suggests the ketogenic diet could play a role in reducing symptoms of depression by improving brain energy metabolism and reducing oxidative stress.

- **Considerations and Challenges:**
- **Adaptation Period:** Transitioning to ketosis can be challenging, with some experiencing the "keto flu," a collection of symptoms like fatigue and brain fog during the initial adaptation period.
- **Sustainability:** Long-term adherence to the ketogenic diet requires careful planning and can be difficult due to its restrictive nature, especially in social situations.
- **Nutritional Deficiencies:** The exclusion of certain food groups may lead to deficiencies in fiber, vitamins, and minerals, necessitating supplementation and mindful meal planning.

II. <u>Intermittent Fasting: Effects on Mental and Emotional Health:</u>

Intermittent fasting (IF) is an eating pattern that alternates between periods of eating and fasting. This approach to eating has been linked to various mental health benefits.

- **Mechanisms of Action:**
- **Autophagy:** Fasting promotes autophagy, a cellular repair process that is beneficial for brain health by clearing out damaged cells and proteins that could contribute to neurodegenerative diseases.
- **Improved Insulin Sensitivity:** IF helps stabilize blood sugar levels, reducing the risk of mood swings and metabolic-related mental health disorders.
- **BDNF Levels:** Fasting increases brain-derived neurotrophic factor (BDNF), which supports neuron growth and resilience, enhancing cognitive function and emotional stability.

- **Mental Health Benefits:**
- **Cognitive Enhancement:** Intermittent fasting has been associated with improved memory, focus, and cognitive resilience, potentially due to increased neurogenesis and reduced inflammation.
- **Mood Regulation:** The stabilization of blood sugar and increased BDNF can lead to more balanced moods and a reduction in symptoms of depression and anxiety.
- **Stress Resistance:** IF may improve the body's stress response by increasing the production of stress-resilient proteins and reducing systemic inflammation.

- **Considerations and Challenges:**
- **Hunger Management:** Managing hunger and irritability during fasting periods can be challenging, especially when first adopting the practice.
- **Risk of Disordered Eating:** For some, intermittent fasting may trigger disordered eating patterns, particularly in those with a history of eating disorders.
- **Suitability:** IF is not suitable for everyone, particularly those with certain health conditions, and should be approached with caution under medical supervision.

III. <u>Gluten-Free Diets: Advantages for Mental Health:</u>

A gluten-free diet is essential for individuals with celiac disease and has been adopted by others for its perceived mental health benefits, particularly in those with non-celiac gluten sensitivity (NCGS).

- **Mechanisms of Action:**
- **Neuroinflammation:** In individuals with gluten sensitivity, consuming gluten can trigger neuroinflammation, leading to symptoms such as brain fog, anxiety, and depression.
- **Gut-Brain Axis:** Gluten can disrupt the gut microbiota, affecting the gut-brain axis and contributing to mood and cognitive issues through inflammatory and immune responses.
- **Nutrient Absorption:** For those with celiac disease or NCGS, gluten consumption impairs nutrient absorption, leading to deficiencies in key nutrients essential for brain health.

- **Mental Health Benefits:**
- **Autism Spectrum Disorders (ASD):** Some evidence suggests that a gluten-free diet may help improve behavioral and cognitive symptoms in individuals with ASD, though research is mixed.
- **Mood Improvement:** Adopting a gluten-free diet can lead to significant improvements in mood and cognitive function for those with gluten sensitivity, reducing symptoms of anxiety and depression.
- **Cognitive Function:** Many individuals with gluten sensitivity report improvements in mental clarity and a reduction in brain fog after eliminating gluten from their diet.

- **Considerations and Challenges:**
- **Nutritional Deficiencies:** A gluten-free diet can lead to deficiencies in fiber, B vitamins, iron, and magnesium, requiring careful dietary planning or supplementation.
- **Social Challenges:** Adhering to a gluten-free diet can be socially challenging, with risks of cross-contamination and limited options when dining out.
- **Cost and Accessibility:** Gluten-free products are often more expensive and less accessible, making the diet challenging for some to maintain.

Conclusion:

Special diets like the ketogenic diet, intermittent fasting, and gluten-free diets offer promising potential for improving mental health by leveraging the power of nutrition to enhance cognitive function, stabilize mood, and protect brain health. However, these diets come with challenges that require careful consideration, including nutritional deficiencies, social limitations, and the need for long-term adherence.

In this chapter, we've explored the mechanisms through which these diets may influence mental health, discussed the benefits and challenges associated with each, and provided practical guidance for those considering these dietary approaches. While the evidence supporting the mental health benefits of these diets is growing, it's essential to approach them with a balanced perspective, recognizing that what works for one individual may not be suitable for another .

As with any dietary change, it's crucial to consult with a healthcare professional to ensure that any special diet is appropriate for your individual health needs and to avoid potential risks. By understanding the connection between diet and mental health, we can make informed choices that support our mental and emotional well-being, leading to a healthier, more balanced life.

Chapter 16
Food Sensitivities and Their Hidden Effects on Mood and Cognition

Sometimes, the problem isn't what you're missing, but what your body is quietly reacting to every day.

I. <u>Identifying and Managing Food Allergies:</u>

Food allergies and sensitivities significantly impact mental health, often in ways that are not immediately apparent. Proper identification and management of these allergies can lead to substantial improvements in both emotional and cognitive well-being.

- **Identifying Food Allergies:**

Food allergies manifest through a range of symptoms, some of which directly affect mental health. Common physical symptoms include digestive issues (such as bloating, diarrhea, and constipation), skin reactions (like rashes, hives, and eczema), and respiratory problems (such as asthma and nasal congestion). However, food allergies can also cause mental health symptoms such as brain fog, anxiety, depression, irritability, and mood swings.

- **Diagnostic Tools:**

To accurately identify food allergies, several diagnostic tools and methods are available:

- **Skin Prick Tests:** A small amount of a suspected allergen is placed on the skin, which is then lightly pricked. A reaction, such as redness or swelling, indicates an allergy.

- **Blood Tests:** These tests measure specific antibodies (IgE) in the blood that are produced in response to allergens.
- **Elimination Diets:** This method involves removing suspected allergens from the diet for a period and then gradually reintroducing them while monitoring for symptoms.

- **Managing Food Allergies:**

Effective management of food allergies is crucial for maintaining mental health. Key strategies include:

- **Avoiding Triggers:** Once identified, avoiding foods that trigger allergic reactions is the most effective way to manage food allergies.
- **Reading Labels:** Learning to read food labels carefully helps prevent accidental exposure to allergens.
- **Substitutes:** Finding suitable substitutes for allergenic foods ensures that nutritional needs are still met without causing adverse reactions.

II. <u>Elimination Diets:</u>

Elimination diets are a powerful tool for identifying food sensitivities that may not present as obvious allergies but still significantly affect mental health.

- **Step-by-Step Guide:**

1 .**Preparation:** Begin by keeping a detailed food diary to track what you eat and any symptoms you experience. This helps identify patterns and potential triggers.

2 .**Elimination Phase:** Remove all potential allergenic foods from your diet for 2-4 weeks. Common allergens include dairy, gluten, soy, nuts,

and eggs. This phase allows the body to clear itself of these substances and reset.

3 .**Reintroduction Phase:** Gradually reintroduce one food at a time every 3-5 days, noting any physical or mental health changes. This helps identify which foods are causing adverse reactions.

4 .**Observation:** Monitor and document your reactions to each food. Symptoms like fatigue, mood changes, digestive issues, and mental clarity can indicate sensitivities.

III.   <u>Case Studies:</u>

- **Real-life case studies illustrate the profound impact elimination diets can have:**
- **Case Study 1:** An individual with chronic anxiety and brain fog discovered a sensitivity to gluten through an elimination diet. Removing gluten from their diet resulted in significant improvements in mental clarity and reduced anxiety.
- **Case Study 2:** A person suffering from persistent fatigue and depression identified dairy as a trigger. Eliminating dairy from their diet led to increased energy levels and a more stable mood.

- **Food Sensitivities and Mental Health:**

Food sensitivities can subtly influence mental health, often going unnoticed and being misattributed to other causes.

o Understanding the Mechanism:

When the body reacts negatively to certain foods, it can trigger inflammation and immune responses. This inflammation can affect the brain, leading to symptoms such as anxiety, depression, brain fog, and cognitive impairments. Unlike food allergies, which involve an immediate immune response, food sensitivities can cause delayed reactions, making them harder to identify.

- **Common Culprits:**
  - **Several common foods are known to cause sensitivities that impact mental health:**
- **Gluten:** Found in wheat, barley, and rye, gluten sensitivity can cause neurological symptoms, including brain fog, headaches, and mood disorders.
- **Dairy:** Lactose intolerance and casein sensitivity in dairy products can lead to digestive issues, mood swings, and cognitive problems.
- **Soy:** Soy can affect hormone levels, potentially impacting mood and mental clarity.
- **Processed Foods:** Additives, preservatives, and artificial colors can trigger sensitivities that affect mental health, contributing to symptoms like hyperactivity, anxiety, and irritability.

  - **Managing Sensitivities:**
- **Personalized Diet Plans:** Working with a healthcare professional to create a diet plan tailored to individual sensitivities can lead to significant improvements in mental health.
- **Mindful Eating:** Paying attention to how foods affect your mood and mental state can help identify problematic foods and promote better dietary choices.

- **Case Studies: Real-Life Examples:**

Real-life examples highlight the profound impact of identifying and managing food allergies and sensitivities on mental health.

- o **Case Study 1: Gluten Sensitivity and Depression**

A young woman experienced chronic depression and fatigue. Traditional treatments offered limited relief. Through an elimination diet, she discovered a sensitivity to gluten. Upon removing gluten from her diet, her symptoms dramatically improved, showcasing the potential of dietary interventions in mental health.

- o **Case Study 2: Dairy and Anxiety**

A middle-aged man suffered from severe anxiety and digestive issues. After eliminating dairy from his diet, his anxiety levels dropped, and his overall well-being improved. This case emphasizes the potential of dietary changes in managing mental health conditions.

- o **Case Study 3: Processed Foods and ADHD**

A child diagnosed with ADHD showed considerable behavioral improvements after eliminating processed foods and artificial additives from his diet. His attention span and academic performance improved, highlighting the role of diet in managing neurodevelopmental disorders.

Conclusion:

Understanding and addressing food allergies and sensitivities can have a transformative effect on mental health. By identifying triggers through careful observation and diagnostic tools, individuals can make informed dietary choices that support their emotional and cognitive well-being. The real-life case studies presented in this chapter illustrate the profound impact dietary changes can have on mental health, encouraging readers to explore and implement these strategies for themselves or their patients. Embracing the connection between diet and mental health empowers individuals to take control of their well-being, fostering a healthier, happier life.

Chapter 17
How Nutritional Needs Change
Across Different Stages of Life

The way you eat can be just as important as what you eat, and often, it shapes your mental state in subtle ways.

I.   <u>Children and Adolescents:</u>

Understanding the unique nutritional needs of children and adolescents is crucial for supporting their mental and behavioral development. This period of rapid growth and development requires a balanced diet to promote healthy physical and cognitive growth.

- **Nutritional Needs for Children:**
- **Proteins:** Essential for building neuronal cells and tissues.
- **Carbohydrates:** Provide the energy needed for physical activity and mental tasks.
- **Healthy Fats:** Support brain development and function.
- **Vitamins and Minerals:** Play a role in nervous system function and mood regulation.
  - **Impact on Behavior and Learning:**
- **Behavior:** Proper nutrition can improve behavior and reduce issues like hyperactivity and irritability.
- **Learning:** Adequate nutrient intake enhances concentration, memory, and overall cognitive performance.
  - **Common Nutritional Deficiencies:**
- **Iron Deficiency:** Can lead to fatigue, irritability, and cognitive impairments.

- **Omega-3 Fatty Acids Deficiency:** Associated with attention deficits and behavioral issues.
- **Vitamin D Deficiency:** Linked to mood disorders such as depression.
  - o **Dietary Recommendations:**
- **Balanced Diet:** Ensure a mix of proteins, carbohydrates, and healthy fats.
- **Whole Foods:** Prioritize whole, unprocessed foods over processed snacks.
- **Hydration:** Maintain adequate hydration to support cognitive function.

II. <u>Adults:</u>

Maintaining mental health during adulthood requires attention to dietary habits that support sustained energy levels, mood stability, and cognitive function.

- o **Nutritional Strategies for Adults:**
- **Balanced Macronutrients:** Consuming balanced proportions of proteins, fats, and carbohydrates.
- **Micronutrient Intake:** Ensuring sufficient intake of vitamins and minerals, such as B vitamins, magnesium, and zinc.
- **Antioxidant-Rich Foods:** Including fruits and vegetables that combat oxidative stress and inflammation.
  - o **Impact of Diet on Stress and Mood:**
- **Stress Management:** Foods rich in magnesium and B vitamins can help manage stress levels.
- **Mood Stabilization:** Omega-3 fatty acids and probiotics support mood regulation and reduce anxiety.
  - o **Common Dietary Challenges:**
- **Busy Lifestyles:** Leading to reliance on fast food and processed meals.

- **Work Stress:** Resulting in emotional eating and poor dietary choices.
  - o **Solutions and Tips:**
- **Meal Planning:** Preparing meals in advance to ensure healthy choices.
- **Mindful Eating:** Paying attention to hunger and fullness cues to avoid overeating.
- **Healthy Snacking:** Keeping nutritious snacks available to prevent unhealthy eating habits.

III.   Seniors:

Addressing the nutritional needs of older adults is essential to support cognitive function and emotional well-being. As the body ages, nutritional requirements and the ability to absorb nutrients change, making dietary considerations even more critical.

  - o **Nutritional Needs for Seniors:**
- **Protein:** Important for maintaining muscle mass and cognitive function.
- **Fiber:** Aids in digestion and prevents constipation.
- **Calcium and Vitamin D:** Essential for bone health and reducing the risk of osteoporosis.
  - o **Impact on Cognitive Health:**
- **Cognitive Decline:** Adequate nutrition can slow down cognitive decline and support brain health.
- **Memory and Concentration:** Nutrients like omega-3 fatty acids, antioxidants, and vitamins B6 and B12 are vital for memory and cognitive function.

o **Common Challenges:**
- **Decreased Appetite:** Seniors often experience a reduced appetite, leading to nutritional deficiencies.
- **Medication Interactions:** Certain medications can affect nutrient absorption and utilization.
  o **Dietary Strategies:**
- **Small, Frequent Meals:** Encouraging smaller, more frequent meals to ensure adequate nutrient intake.
- **Nutrient-Dense Foods:** Focusing on nutrient-dense foods to maximize the intake of essential vitamins and minerals.
- **Hydration:** Ensuring adequate fluid intake to prevent dehydration, which can affect cognitive function.

Conclusion:

Nutritional psychiatry across different age groups highlights the importance of tailored dietary interventions to support mental health. From children and adolescents to adults and seniors, each stage of life has unique nutritional needs that must be addressed to promote optimal cognitive and emotional well-being. By understanding and implementing these age-specific dietary strategies, individuals and clinicians can foster better mental health outcomes, encouraging a healthier, more balanced life at every age.

Chapter 18
Mindful Eating: Rewiring Your Relationship with Food and Mental Health

The way you eat can be just as important as what you eat, and often, it shapes your mental state in subtle ways.

I. <u>The Concept of Mindful Eating:</u>

Mindful eating is an approach that emphasizes awareness and presence during meals. It involves paying attention to the sensory experience of eating, recognizing hunger and fullness cues, and fostering a non-judgmental attitude towards food.

- **Definition and Principles:**
- **Awareness:** Being fully present and attentive to the eating experience.
- **Non-Judgment:** Avoiding labeling foods as "good" or "bad".
- **Sensory Focus:** Engaging all senses to appreciate the colors, textures, smells, and flavors of food.
- **Recognition of Hunger and Fullness:** Listening to the body's signals to eat when hungry and stop when full.

- **Benefits of Mindful Eating:**
- **Reduced Overeating:** By paying attention to hunger and fullness cues, mindful eating can help prevent overeating.
- **Improved Digestion:** Eating slowly and mindfully can enhance digestion and nutrient absorption.
- **Enhanced Enjoyment:** Fully experiencing the flavors and textures of food can increase enjoyment and satisfaction from meals.

II. **Practices for Mindful Eating:**

Incorporating mindful eating into daily life involves simple, practical steps that can transform the eating experience.

- **Step-by-Step Guide:**

1 .**Create a Calm Eating Environment:** Minimize distractions such as TV, phones, and computers during meals.

2 .**Take Small Bites:** Focus on taking smaller bites and chewing thoroughly to savor each mouthful.

3 .**Pause Between Bites:** Put down utensils between bites to slow down the eating process and give your body time to register fullness.

4 .**Engage the Senses:** Notice the colors, smells, tastes, and textures of your food.

5 .**Listen to Your Body:** Pay attention to signals of hunger and fullness, eating until you feel satisfied, not stuffed.

6 .**Express Gratitude:** Take a moment to appreciate the food and the effort that went into preparing it.

- **Daily Practices:**
- **Mindful Snacking:** Apply the same principles of mindful eating to snacks, choosing healthier options and savoring them.
- **Mindful Cooking:** Engage in the cooking process by focusing on the ingredients, smells, and textures as you prepare meals.

III. <u>Benefits of Mindful Eating:</u>

Mindful eating has profound effects on mental health, offering numerous psychological and emotional benefits.

- **Reduced Stress and Anxiety:**
- **Focus and Calm:** The practice of mindful eating can create a sense of calm and focus, reducing stress and anxiety levels.
- **Emotional Regulation:** By promoting awareness of emotions related to food, mindful eating can help manage emotional eating and improve emotional regulation.

- **Improved Self-Esteem and Body Image:**
- **Positive Relationship with Food:** Mindful eating encourages a healthier, more positive relationship with food, reducing guilt and shame associated with eating.
- **Body Awareness:** Increased awareness of body signals can lead to a more positive body image and self-esteem.

- **Enhanced Cognitive Function:**
- **Mental Clarity:** By reducing distractions and focusing on the eating experience, mindful eating can enhance mental clarity and concentration.
- **Better Decision-Making:** Improved awareness and presence can lead to better food choices and overall decision-making.

- **Case Studies: Real-Life Applications:**

Real-life examples illustrate the transformative impact of mindful eating on mental health and overall well-being.

- o **Case Study 1: Overcoming Emotional Eating**

A woman struggling with emotional eating found solace in mindful eating practices. By recognizing her emotional triggers and focusing on the sensory experience of eating, she was able to manage her emotional eating, leading to improved mood and self-esteem.

- o **Case Study 2: Reducing Anxiety**

A man with high levels of anxiety started practicing mindful eating as a part of his daily routine. He reported a significant reduction in anxiety levels, better digestion, and a more positive relationship with food.

- o **Case Study 3: Enhancing Cognitive Performance**

A student struggling with concentration and cognitive performance began incorporating mindful eating into her study routine. By slowing down and savoring her meals, she noticed improved focus, better retention of information, and reduced stress.

Conclusion:

Mindful eating is a powerful tool for enhancing mental health and overall well-being. By fostering a deeper connection with the eating experience, individuals can improve their relationship with food, reduce stress and anxiety, and enhance cognitive function. The practical steps and real-life examples provided in this chapter demonstrate the profound impact mindful eating can have, encouraging readers to incorporate these practices into their daily lives for better mental and physical health.

Chapter 19
Supplements and Mental Health:
What Works, What Doesn't, and Why

In a world full of promises and pills, knowing what truly helps, and what doesn't can make all the difference.

I.   <u>Common Supplements:</u>

Supplements can play a crucial role in supporting mental health by filling nutritional gaps and providing specific nutrients that may be lacking in the diet. Understanding which supplements are beneficial for mental well-being is essential for both individuals and healthcare providers.

- **Overview of Key Supplements:**
- **Omega-3 Fatty Acids:** Found in fish oil, these are essential for brain health and have been shown to reduce symptoms of depression and anxiety.
- **B Vitamins:** Including B6, B12, and folate, these vitamins are vital for energy production and neurotransmitter synthesis, which can influence mood and cognitive function.
- **Vitamin D:** Often referred to as the "sunshine vitamin," it plays a role in mood regulation and has been linked to reduced symptoms of depression.
- **Magnesium:** Known for its calming effects, magnesium can help manage stress and improve sleep quality.
- **Zinc:** This mineral is important for brain function and has been associated with reduced symptoms of depression and anxiety.

- **Benefits and Uses:**

- **Mood Stabilization:** Supplements like omega-3 fatty acids and B vitamins can help stabilize mood and reduce mood swings.
- **Cognitive Enhancement:** Vitamins and minerals such as B12, magnesium, and zinc support cognitive functions like memory, focus, and mental clarity.
- **Stress Reduction:** Magnesium and omega-3s are known for their stress-reducing properties, helping individuals manage daily stressors more effectively.

II.   <u>Herbal Supplements:</u>

Herbal supplements have been used for centuries to support mental health. Many herbs have scientifically proven benefits for reducing anxiety, improving mood, and enhancing overall well-being.

- **Popular Herbal Supplements:**

- **St. John's Wort:** Commonly used for mild to moderate depression, this herb has antidepressant properties due to its active compounds like hypericin and hyperforin.
- **Valerian Root:** Known for its calming effects, valerian root can help improve sleep quality and reduce anxiety.
- **Ashwagandha:** An adaptogen that helps the body manage stress, ashwagandha can improve overall mental health and reduce symptoms of anxiety and depression.
- **Rhodiola Rosea:** This adaptogen can enhance mental performance, reduce fatigue, and improve resilience to stress.

- **Mechanisms of Action:**
- **Neurotransmitter Modulation:** Many herbal supplements influence the levels of neurotransmitters like serotonin, dopamine, and GABA, which are crucial for mood regulation.
- **Anti-Inflammatory Effects:** Some herbs have anti-inflammatory properties that can reduce inflammation in the brain, which is linked to mental health disorders.
- **Antioxidant Properties:** Herbs like Rhodiola Rosea have antioxidant effects that protect brain cells from oxidative stress and improve overall brain health.

III. <u>Choosing the Right Supplements:</u>

Selecting the appropriate supplements for mental health involves understanding individual needs, potential interactions, and the quality of the supplements.

- **Guidelines for Selection:**
- **Consult with a Healthcare Provider:** Always consult a healthcare professional before starting any supplement regimen to ensure safety and appropriateness.
- **Quality and Purity:** Choose supplements from reputable brands that undergo third-party testing for quality and purity.
- **Dosage and Timing:** Follow recommended dosages and consider the timing of supplements for optimal absorption and effectiveness.

- **Potential Interactions and Side Effects:**
- **Drug Interactions:** Some supplements can interact with medications, so it's important to discuss with a healthcare provider to avoid adverse effects.

- **Side Effects:** Be aware of possible side effects, such as gastrointestinal discomfort or allergic reactions, and discontinue use if any adverse symptoms occur.

- **Case Studies:**
- **Managing Depression with Omega-3s:** A patient with moderate depression experienced significant improvement in mood and cognitive function after incorporating omega-3 supplements into their diet.
- **Reducing Anxiety with Ashwagandha:** A person suffering from chronic anxiety reported reduced symptoms and improved stress management after using ashwagandha regularly.

Conclusion:

Supplements can be a valuable addition to a holistic approach to mental health, offering benefits for mood stabilization, cognitive enhancement, and stress reduction. By understanding the role of different supplements and choosing them wisely, individuals can support their mental well-being effectively. However, it is crucial to consult healthcare professionals and consider quality and safety when incorporating supplements into a mental health regimen. This chapter provides a comprehensive guide to the most beneficial supplements for mental health, encouraging readers to make informed choices for their well-being.

Chapter 20
How Culture and Society Shape the Way We Eat, and Think

Your food choices are rarely just personal, they are influenced by a much larger system you may not even notice.

I. Cultural Dietary Practices:

Dietary habits and preferences are deeply rooted in cultural traditions and practices. These cultural dietary practices can significantly impact mental health, either positively or negatively.

- **Traditional Diets:**
- **Mediterranean Diet:** Rich in fruits, vegetables, whole grains, and healthy fats, this diet is associated with lower rates of depression and cognitive decline.
- **Japanese Diet:** High in fish, vegetables, and fermented foods, this diet supports mental health through its nutrient-dense and anti-inflammatory properties.
- **Indian Diet:** Featuring spices like turmeric and a variety of plant-based foods, the Indian diet has components that support brain health and reduce inflammation.

- **Positive Impacts on Mental Health:**
- **Nutrient Density:** Traditional diets are often rich in essential nutrients that support brain function and mental health.

- **Anti-Inflammatory Foods:** Many traditional diets include foods with anti-inflammatory properties, which can help reduce the risk of mental health disorders.

- **Negative Impacts:**
- **High Carbohydrate Intake:** Some cultural diets may include high amounts of refined carbohydrates, which can negatively impact mood and energy levels.
- **Cultural Resistance to Change:** Cultural attachment to certain unhealthy foods can make it challenging to adopt healthier eating habits.

II. <u>Societal Changes:</u>

Modern societal changes have significantly altered dietary patterns, often leading to negative consequences for mental health.

- **Impact of Processed Foods:**
- **High Sugar and Fat Content:** The increased consumption of processed foods high in sugar and unhealthy fats is linked to higher rates of depression and anxiety.
- **Nutrient Deficiency:** Processed foods are often low in essential nutrients, contributing to deficiencies that can affect mental health.

- **Fast-Paced Lifestyles:**
- **Convenience Foods:** The reliance on fast and convenience foods due to busy lifestyles often leads to poor dietary choices.
- **Irregular Eating Patterns:** Skipping meals or eating at irregular times can disrupt blood sugar levels and impact mood and cognitive function.

- **Urbanization and Mental Health:**
- **Reduced Access to Fresh Foods:** Urban environments may limit access to fresh, healthy foods, leading to higher consumption of processed and fast foods.
- **Social Isolation:** Urban living can increase social isolation, which is linked to poor mental health outcomes.

III.   Promoting Healthy Eating in Communities:

Addressing the challenges posed by cultural and societal influences requires community-wide efforts to promote healthy eating habits.

- **Community Programs and Initiatives:**
- **Educational Campaigns:** Programs that educate communities about the importance of nutrition for mental health can encourage healthier eating habits.
- **Community Gardens:** Initiatives that promote community gardening can increase access to fresh, nutritious foods and foster a sense of community.
- **Local Farmers' Markets:** Supporting local farmers' markets can provide communities with access to fresh, locally grown produce.

- **Policy Changes:**
- **Nutrition Education in Schools:** Implementing comprehensive nutrition education in schools can instill healthy eating habits from a young age.
- **Subsidies for Healthy Foods:** Policies that subsidize healthy foods and reduce the cost of fresh produce can make healthier options more accessible to everyone.

- **Collaboration with Cultural Leaders:**
- **Engaging Cultural Leaders:** Working with cultural leaders to promote healthy dietary changes can help bridge the gap between tradition and modern health recommendations.
- **Culturally Sensitive Approaches:** Tailoring health messages to respect and incorporate cultural practices can enhance acceptance and effectiveness.

Conclusion:

Cultural and societal influences play a significant role in shaping dietary habits and, consequently, mental health. By understanding and addressing these influences, communities can promote healthier eating patterns that support mental well-being. This chapter highlights the importance of considering cultural practices and societal changes in efforts to improve nutrition and mental health. Through education, community initiatives, and policy changes, it is possible to foster environments that encourage and support healthy eating habits, ultimately benefiting mental health on a broader scale.

Chapter 21
The Next Frontier: Personalized Nutrition and Mental Health Innovation

The future of mental health may not be one-size-fits-all, but tailored precisely to your unique biology.

I. Advances in Nutritional Research:

The field of nutritional psychiatry is rapidly evolving, with ongoing research uncovering new insights into how diet impacts mental health. Several emerging trends are shaping the future of this field.

- **Microbiome Research:**
  - **Gut-Brain Axis:** Understanding the complex communication between the gut microbiome and the brain is a major focus. Research is exploring how gut bacteria influence mood, cognition, and behavior.
  - **Probiotics and Prebiotics:** Studies are examining the potential of probiotics and prebiotics to improve mental health by modulating the gut microbiome.

- **Nutrigenomics:**
  - **Personalized Nutrition:** Nutrigenomics, the study of how genes interact with diet, is paving the way for personalized nutrition plans tailored to individual genetic profiles.

- **Gene-Diet Interactions:** Research is identifying specific genetic variations that affect how individuals respond to different nutrients, which can inform targeted dietary interventions for mental health.

- **Anti-Inflammatory Diets:**
- **Inflammation and Mental Health:** Chronic inflammation is linked to various mental health disorders. Diets rich in anti-inflammatory foods are being studied for their potential to reduce inflammation and improve mental health.
- **Omega-3 Fatty Acids:** The role of omega-3 fatty acids in reducing inflammation and supporting brain health continues to be a significant area of research.

II. <u>Innovative Therapies:</u>

New and innovative nutritional therapies are being developed to address mental health challenges more effectively.

- **Nutritional Supplements:**
- **Advanced Formulations:** Researchers are developing advanced supplement formulations that combine multiple nutrients to support mental health synergistically.
- **Targeted Supplements:** Specific supplements targeting neurotransmitter production, inflammation, and oxidative stress are being explored for their potential benefits.

- **Functional Foods:**
- **Fortified Foods:** Foods fortified with vitamins, minerals, and other bioactive compounds are being designed to support mental health.

- **Adaptogenic Foods:** Incorporating adaptogens like ashwagandha and Rhodiola Rosea into functional foods to help manage stress and improve mental resilience.

- **Dietary Protocols:**
- **Elimination Diets:** Personalized elimination diets are used to identify and remove foods that may negatively impact mental health.
- **Timed Eating:** Exploring the benefits of meal timing and fasting protocols on mental health and cognitive function.

III.   <u>Research Opportunities:</u>

Despite the progress, many areas within nutritional psychiatry require further exploration.

- **Longitudinal Studies:**
- **Long-Term Effects:** More long-term studies are needed to understand the sustained impact of dietary interventions on mental health.
- **Diverse Populations:** Research should include diverse populations to understand how cultural, genetic, and environmental factors influence the effectiveness of nutritional interventions.

- **Mechanistic Studies:**
- **Biological Pathways:** Investigating the specific biological pathways through which nutrients affect brain function and mental health.
- **Microbiome Mechanisms:** Detailed studies on how changes in the gut microbiome translate to changes in mental health outcomes.

- **Clinical Trials:**
- **Standardized Protocols:** Developing standardized protocols for clinical trials to ensure consistency and comparability of results.
- **Combination Therapies:** Exploring the combined effects of diet, supplements, and other lifestyle interventions on mental health.

IV. **Personalized Nutrition:**

Personalized nutrition represents a promising frontier in nutritional psychiatry, offering customized dietary recommendations based on individual characteristics.

- **Genetic Profiling:**
- **DNA Testing:** Using DNA testing to identify genetic predispositions that affect nutrient metabolism and mental health.
- **Customized Diet Plans:** Creating personalized diet plans that cater to an individual's genetic makeup and nutritional needs.

- **Lifestyle Factors:**
- **Holistic Approach:** Considering lifestyle factors such as physical activity, sleep, and stress management in personalized nutrition plans.
- **Integrative Therapies:** Combining personalized nutrition with other therapeutic approaches for a comprehensive mental health strategy.

- **Technological Advancements:**
- **Digital Tools:** Leveraging digital tools and apps to monitor dietary intake, track mental health symptoms, and provide personalized recommendations.

- **Wearable Devices:** Using wearable devices to collect real-time data on physical and mental health, which can inform personalized nutrition strategies.

Conclusion:

The future of nutritional psychiatry is bright, with ongoing research and innovation driving the field forward. Advances in understanding the gut-brain axis, nutrigenomics, and anti-inflammatory diets are opening new avenues for improving mental health through nutrition. Innovative therapies and personalized nutrition plans offer the potential for more effective and tailored interventions. As research continues to evolve, the integration of diet, lifestyle, and technology will play a crucial role in shaping the future of mental health care. This chapter highlights the exciting trends and opportunities in nutritional psychiatry, encouraging readers to stay informed and engaged with this rapidly growing field.

Conclusion

The Role of Nutrition in Mental Health: A Clinical Perspective has taken you on a comprehensive journey through the intricate relationship between nutrition and mental health. Our exploration has underscored the profound impact that dietary choices can have on cognitive function, emotional well-being, and overall mental health. From understanding the role of macronutrients and micronutrients to delving into the gut-brain connection and dietary patterns, we've covered essential topics to equip you with the knowledge needed to make informed decisions for your mental health.

I.   Key Takeaways:

1 .The Importance of Balanced Nutrition:

-   Proper nutrition is fundamental to maintaining optimal brain function and emotional stability. A balanced diet, rich in a variety of nutrients, provides the building blocks for neurotransmitter production, hormonal balance, and overall brain health. Essential fatty acids, amino acids, vitamins, and minerals all play crucial roles in these processes.

2 .Macronutrients and Mental Health:

-   **Proteins:** Amino acids, the building blocks of proteins, are vital for the synthesis of neurotransmitters such as serotonin, dopamine, and norepinephrine. Adequate protein intake ensures that the brain has the necessary components to maintain mood stability and cognitive function.
-   **Carbohydrates:** Carbohydrates are the brain's primary source of energy. Complex carbohydrates, in particular, provide a steady supply

of glucose, preventing the blood sugar spikes and crashes that can affect mood and energy levels. Additionally, carbohydrates are involved in the production of serotonin, a key neurotransmitter for mood regulation.

- **Fats:** Healthy fats, especially omega-3 fatty acids, are integral to brain health. They contribute to the structural integrity of brain cells and play a role in reducing inflammation, which is linked to various mental health conditions.

3 .Micronutrients Matter:

- **Vitamins:** Vitamins such as B12, B6, folate, and vitamin D are essential for brain function. B vitamins are involved in neurotransmitter synthesis and nerve function, while vitamin D has been shown to affect mood and cognitive function.
- **Minerals:** Minerals like magnesium, zinc, and iron are crucial for mental health. Magnesium is involved in over 300 biochemical reactions, including those that regulate mood. Zinc plays a role in neurotransmitter function and neuroplasticity, and iron is essential for oxygen transport in the brain.

4 .The Gut-Brain Axis:

- The connection between the gut and the brain is a pivotal area of study in nutritional psychiatry. The gut microbiome, which consists of trillions of microorganisms, communicates with the brain via the vagus nerve and through the production of neurotransmitters and other signaling molecules. A healthy gut microbiome, supported by a diet rich in fiber, probiotics, and prebiotics, can positively influence mental health by reducing inflammation and supporting the production of mood-regulating neurotransmitters.

5 .Dietary Patterns and Their Impacts:

- **Mediterranean Diet:** This diet, rich in fruits, vegetables, whole grains, nuts, and healthy fats, has been associated with a lower risk of depression and cognitive decline. The Mediterranean diet provides a broad range of nutrients that support brain health and reduce inflammation.
- **Plant-Based Diets:** Vegetarian and vegan diets, when well-planned, can provide all the necessary nutrients for mental health. These diets emphasize nutrient-dense foods that are high in antioxidants, vitamins, and minerals.
- **Western Diet:** Diets high in processed foods, sugars, and unhealthy fats are linked to an increased risk of mental health issues such as depression and anxiety. These diets often lack essential nutrients and contribute to inflammation and oxidative stress.

6 .Targeted Nutritional Interventions:

- **For Depression:** Diets rich in omega-3 fatty acids, B vitamins, and antioxidants can help alleviate symptoms of depression. Foods such as fatty fish, leafy greens, and berries are particularly beneficial.
- **For Anxiety:** Magnesium-rich foods, probiotics, and herbal teas can help reduce anxiety. Incorporating foods like nuts, seeds, yogurt, and chamomile tea into the diet can have calming effects.
- **For Neurodevelopmental Disorders:** Nutritional strategies for conditions such as ADHD and autism include ensuring adequate intake of omega-3 fatty acids, iron, zinc, and other essential nutrients. Personalized dietary plans can help manage symptoms and improve quality of life for individuals with these conditions.

7 .Practical Application in Clinical Practice:

- **Assessment:** Clinicians should conduct comprehensive nutritional assessments to identify deficiencies and dietary habits that may impact mental health. This includes reviewing medical history, lifestyle factors, and conducting blood tests if necessary.
- **Personalized Plans:** Developing individualized dietary plans that address specific nutritional needs and preferences is crucial. Collaborating with dietitians and nutritionists can enhance the effectiveness of these plans.
- **Monitoring and Adjustment:** Regular follow-up appointments to monitor progress and adjust dietary plans as needed are essential for achieving long-term success. Clinicians should be prepared to address challenges such as financial constraints, psychological resistance, and cultural preferences.

II.   Looking Ahead:

The field of nutritional psychiatry is rapidly evolving, with ongoing research uncovering new insights into how diet affects mental health. Future directions may include:

- **Personalized Nutrition:** Advances in genetics and microbiome research may lead to more personalized dietary recommendations based on individual needs.
- **Nutritional Therapies:** Developing new nutritional therapies and supplements to target specific mental health conditions.
- **Integration into Healthcare:** Increasing the integration of nutritional approaches into mainstream mental health care, supported by comprehensive training for clinicians and collaboration across disciplines.

III.   <u>Final Thoughts:</u>

Your journey through this book has provided a solid foundation in understanding the crucial role of nutrition in mental health. By applying the knowledge and strategies discussed, you can make more informed choices that support both your physical and mental well-being. Whether you are a clinician aiming to enhance your practice or an individual seeking to improve your mental health, the principles outlined in this book offer valuable guidance for achieving better mental health through nutrition.

Remember, the path to mental wellness is multifaceted, and nutrition is a powerful tool that, when combined with other therapeutic approaches, can lead to significant improvements in mental health. Continue to educate yourself, stay curious, and prioritize your health through mindful and informed dietary choices..

Results

After an extensive exploration of the role of nutrition in mental health, several key findings highlight the significant impact dietary choices can have on cognitive function, emotional well-being, and overall mental health. These findings are based on scientific research, clinical practices, and practical experiences.

1. Balanced Nutrition is Essential for Optimal Mental Health:

- **Nutrient Diversity:**

  - A balanced diet that includes a variety of nutrients is crucial for maintaining brain health and emotional stability. Essential fatty acids, amino acids, vitamins, and minerals all contribute significantly to the synthesis and function of neurotransmitters and hormones that regulate mood and cognition.
  - **Proteins:** Amino acids from protein are essential for the production of neurotransmitters. Tryptophan, for example, is necessary for serotonin production, which influences mood, sleep, and appetite.
  - **Healthy Fats:** Omega-3 fatty acids, found in fish, flaxseeds, and walnuts, are crucial for brain health. They support the structural integrity of brain cells and have anti-inflammatory properties that protect against depression and anxiety.

- **Energy Supply:**

  - The brain relies on a consistent and adequate supply of energy, primarily from carbohydrates. Complex carbohydrates, such as whole grains and vegetables, provide a steady release of glucose, preventing

blood sugar spikes and crashes that can lead to mood swings and cognitive impairments.
- **Fiber-Rich Foods:** High-fiber foods help stabilize blood sugar levels, reducing the risk of mood swings and providing sustained energy for the brain.

2. Macronutrients and Their Critical Roles:

- **Proteins:**
- Proteins are composed of amino acids, which are essential for the production of neurotransmitters like serotonin, dopamine, and norepinephrine. These neurotransmitters are vital for mood regulation, cognitive function, and overall mental health. Consuming adequate protein ensures that the brain has the necessary components for these processes.
- **Sources of Protein:** Lean meats, fish, eggs, dairy products, legumes, and nuts are excellent sources of high-quality protein.

- **Carbohydrates:**
- Carbohydrates are the primary energy source for the brain. Complex carbohydrates are particularly beneficial as they provide a steady supply of glucose, which helps maintain stable energy levels and mood. Additionally, carbohydrates play a role in the production of serotonin, a neurotransmitter that promotes feelings of well-being and happiness.
- **Whole Grains:** Foods like oats, quinoa, and brown rice are excellent sources of complex carbohydrates and provide long-lasting energy.

- **Fats:**
- Healthy fats, especially omega-3 fatty acids, are crucial for brain health. They contribute to the structural integrity of brain cells and have anti-inflammatory properties. Omega-3 fatty acids, found in fatty fish, flaxseeds, and walnuts, are linked to improved cognitive function and a lower risk of mental health disorders like depression and anxiety.
- **Sources of Healthy Fats:** In addition to fish and nuts, avocados, olive oil, and seeds are great sources of healthy fats.

3. Micronutrients are Vital for Brain Function:

- **Vitamins:**
- Vitamins such as B12, B6, folate, and vitamin D are essential for brain health. B vitamins are involved in neurotransmitter synthesis and nerve function, while vitamin D influences mood and cognitive function. Deficiencies in these vitamins can lead to mental health issues such as depression, fatigue, and cognitive decline.
- **Sources of B Vitamins:** Whole grains, meat, eggs, dairy products, and leafy green vegetables.
- **Sources of Vitamin D:** Sunlight exposure, fatty fish, fortified dairy products, and supplements.

- **Minerals:**
- Minerals like magnesium, zinc, and iron play significant roles in mental health. Magnesium is involved in over 300 biochemical reactions, including those that regulate mood and brain function. Zinc contributes to neuroplasticity and neurotransmitter function, while iron is essential for oxygen transport in the brain. Deficiencies in

these minerals can lead to symptoms like anxiety, depression, and impaired cognitive function.

- **Sources of Magnesium:** Nuts, seeds, whole grains, and green leafy vegetables.
- **Sources of Zinc:** Meat, shellfish, legumes, and seeds.
- **Sources of Iron:** Red meat, beans, lentils, and fortified cereals.

4. The Gut-Brain Axis:

• **Microbiome Communication:**
- The gut microbiome, which consists of trillions of microorganisms, communicates with the brain via the vagus nerve and through the production of neurotransmitters and other signaling molecules. A healthy gut microbiome, supported by a diet rich in fiber, probiotics, and prebiotics, can positively influence mental health by reducing inflammation and supporting the production of mood-regulating neurotransmitters.
- **Probiotics:** Live bacteria that provide health benefits when consumed in adequate amounts. Sources include yogurt, kefir, sauerkraut, and other fermented foods.
- **Prebiotics:** Non-digestible food components that promote the growth of beneficial gut bacteria. Sources include garlic, onions, bananas, and whole grains.

• **Impact on Inflammation:**
- A balanced diet that promotes a healthy gut microbiome can help reduce systemic inflammation, which is linked to various mental health conditions. Foods like fermented vegetables, yogurt, and high-fiber foods such as fruits, vegetables, and whole grains can support a healthy gut microbiome.

- **Anti-Inflammatory Foods:** Berries, fatty fish, leafy greens, and nuts can help reduce inflammation and support overall mental health.

5. Dietary Patterns and Their Impacts on Mental Health:

- **Mediterranean Diet:**
- The Mediterranean diet, rich in fruits, vegetables, whole grains, nuts, and healthy fats like olive oil, has been associated with a lower risk of depression and cognitive decline. This diet provides a wide range of nutrients that support brain health and reduce inflammation.
- **Key Components:** Olive oil, fish, nuts, legumes, whole grains, and a high intake of fruits and vegetables.

- **Plant-Based Diets:**
- Well-planned vegetarian and vegan diets can provide all the necessary nutrients for mental health. These diets emphasize nutrient-dense foods that are high in antioxidants, vitamins, and minerals, which are essential for brain health and emotional stability.
- **Sources of Plant-Based Nutrients:** Beans, lentils, tofu, nuts, seeds, fruits, and vegetables.

- **Western Diet:**
- Diets high in processed foods, sugars, and unhealthy fats are linked to an increased risk of mental health issues such as depression and anxiety. These diets often lack essential nutrients and contribute to inflammation and oxidative stress, which can negatively impact brain function and mood.
- **Avoiding Processed Foods:** Reducing intake of sugary snacks, fast food, and pre-packaged meals in favor of whole, unprocessed foods.

6. Targeted Nutritional Interventions for Mental Health Disorders:

- **For Depression:**
- Diets rich in omega-3 fatty acids, B vitamins, and antioxidants can help alleviate symptoms of depression. Foods such as fatty fish, leafy greens, berries, and nuts are particularly beneficial. Omega-3 fatty acids reduce inflammation, B vitamins support neurotransmitter function, and antioxidants protect brain cells from oxidative stress.
- **Foods to Include:** Salmon, spinach, blueberries, and almonds.

- **For Anxiety:**
- Magnesium-rich foods, probiotics, and herbal teas can help reduce anxiety. Incorporating foods like nuts, seeds, yogurt, and chamomile tea into the diet can have calming effects. Magnesium supports neurotransmitter function, probiotics promote a healthy gut-brain axis, and herbal teas can have soothing properties.
- **Foods to Include:** Pumpkin seeds, Greek yogurt, and chamomile tea.

- **For Neurodevelopmental Disorders:**
- Nutritional strategies for conditions such as ADHD and autism include ensuring adequate intake of omega-3 fatty acids, iron, zinc, and other essential nutrients. Personalized dietary plans that address specific nutritional needs can help manage symptoms and improve the quality of life for individuals with these conditions.
- **Foods to Include:** Sardines, fortified cereals, and beans.

7. Practical Application in Clinical Practice:

- **Assessment:**
- Clinicians should conduct comprehensive nutritional assessments to identify deficiencies and dietary habits that may impact mental health. This includes reviewing medical history, lifestyle factors, and conducting blood tests if necessary.
- **Tools for Assessment:** Dietary questionnaires, food diaries, and blood tests for nutrient levels.

- **Personalized Plans:**
- Developing individualized dietary plans that address specific nutritional needs and preferences is crucial. Collaborating with dietitians and nutritionists can enhance the effectiveness of these plans. Personalized plans should consider factors such as cultural preferences, financial constraints, and individual health conditions.
- **Creating Customized Plans:** Tailoring dietary recommendations to each patient's unique needs and circumstances.

- **Monitoring and Adjustment:**
- Regular follow-up appointments to monitor progress and adjust dietary plans as needed are essential for achieving long-term success. Clinicians should be prepared to address challenges such as psychological resistance, adherence issues, and any new health concerns that may arise.
- **Continuous Support:** Providing ongoing guidance and encouragement to help patients maintain healthy dietary habits.